Public Health: A Very Short Introduction

VERY SHORT INTRODUCTIONS are for anyone wanting a stimulating and accessible way into a new subject. They are written by experts, and have been translated into more than 40 different languages.

The series began in 1995, and now covers a wide variety of topics in every discipline. The VSI library now contains over 450 volumes—a Very Short Introduction to everything from Psychology and Philosophy of Science to American History and Relativity—and continues to grow in every subject area.

Very Short Introductions available now:

ACCOUNTING Christopher Nobes
ADOLESCENCE Peter K. Smith
ADVERTISING Winston Fletcher
AFRICAN AMERICAN RELIGION
    Eddie S. Glaude Jr
AFRICAN HISTORY John Parker
    and Richard Rathbone
AFRICAN RELIGIONS Jacob K. Olupona
AGNOSTICISM Robin Le Poidevin
AGRICULTURE Paul Brassley and
    Richard Soffe
ALEXANDER THE GREAT
    Hugh Bowden
ALGEBRA Peter M. Higgins
AMERICAN HISTORY Paul S. Boyer
AMERICAN IMMIGRATION
    David A. Gerber
AMERICAN LEGAL HISTORY
    G. Edward White
AMERICAN POLITICAL HISTORY
    Donald Critchlow
AMERICAN POLITICAL PARTIES
    AND ELECTIONS L. Sandy Maisel
AMERICAN POLITICS
    Richard M. Valelly
THE AMERICAN PRESIDENCY
    Charles O. Jones
THE AMERICAN REVOLUTION
    Robert J. Allison
AMERICAN SLAVERY
    Heather Andrea Williams
THE AMERICAN WEST Stephen Aron
AMERICAN WOMEN'S HISTORY
    Susan Ware

ANAESTHESIA Aidan O'Donnell
ANARCHISM Colin Ward
ANCIENT ASSYRIA Karen Radner
ANCIENT EGYPT Ian Shaw
ANCIENT EGYPTIAN ART AND
    ARCHITECTURE Christina Riggs
ANCIENT GREECE Paul Cartledge
THE ANCIENT NEAR EAST
    Amanda H. Podany
ANCIENT PHILOSOPHY Julia Annas
ANCIENT WARFARE
    Harry Sidebottom
ANGELS David Albert Jones
ANGLICANISM Mark Chapman
THE ANGLO-SAXON AGE John Blair
THE ANIMAL KINGDOM
    Peter Holland
ANIMAL RIGHTS David DeGrazia
THE ANTARCTIC Klaus Dodds
ANTISEMITISM Steven Beller
ANXIETY Daniel Freeman and
    Jason Freeman
THE APOCRYPHAL GOSPELS
    Paul Foster
ARCHAEOLOGY Paul Bahn
ARCHITECTURE Andrew Ballantyne
ARISTOCRACY William Doyle
ARISTOTLE Jonathan Barnes
ART HISTORY Dana Arnold
ART THEORY Cynthia Freeland
ASTROBIOLOGY David C. Catling
ASTROPHYSICS James Binney
ATHEISM Julian Baggini
AUGUSTINE Henry Chadwick

Available soon:

For more information visit our website

www.oup.com/vsi/

Virginia Berridge

PUBLIC HEALTH

A Very Short Introduction

OXFORD
UNIVERSITY PRESS

OXFORD
UNIVERSITY PRESS

Great Clarendon Street, Oxford, OX2 6DP,
United Kingdom

Oxford University Press is a department of the University of Oxford.
It furthers the University's objective of excellence in research, scholarship,
and education by publishing worldwide. Oxford is a registered trade mark of
Oxford University Press in the UK and in certain other countries

© Virginia Berridge 2016

The moral rights of the author have been asserted

First edition published in 2016

Impression: 1

Published in the United States of America by Oxford University Press
198 Madison Avenue, New York, NY 10016, United States of America

British Library Cataloguing in Publication Data
Data available

Library of Congress Control Number: 2016935483

ISBN 978-0-19-968846-3

Printed in Great Britain by
Ashford Colour Press Ltd, Gosport, Hampshire

Contents

Acknowledgements

I have been teaching the history of public health to public health students throughout my career at the London School of Hygiene and Tropical Medicine and that has helped enormously with this book. The chapters about recent issues have been aided by my observation of the public health scene, from listening to my colleagues' research papers and lectures and from conversations with them. Particular thanks are due to Dr Alan Maryon Davies, Professor David Heymann, and Professor Wayne Hall, who discussed current and future public health issues with me.

Dr Suzanne Taylor helped with checking and with the illustrations, Ingrid James with practical administrative support. My other colleagues at the Centre for History in Public Health have also contributed considerably over time.

November 2015

List of illustrations

List of abbreviations

AIDS	Acquired Immune deficiency syndrome
ASH	Action on Smoking and Health
BSE	Bovine Spongiform Encephalopathy
CMO	Chief Medical Officer
DDT	dichlorodiphenyltrichloroethane
GATT	General Agreement on Tariffs and Trade
GAVI	Global Alliance for Vaccines and Immunisation
GOBI	Growth monitoring, oral rehydration, breast feeding, and immunization
GP	general practitioner
HFA	Health For All
HIV	Human immunodeficiency virus
HPA	Health Protection Agency
ILO	International Labour Organization
LIC	low income country
LNHO	League of Nations Health Organization
MDGs	Millennium Development Goals
MMR	measles, mumps, and rubella
MoH	Medical Officer of Health
MRSA	methicillin-resistant *Staphylococcus aureus*
NCD	non-communicable disease
NGO	non-governmental organization
NICE	National Institute for Health and Care Excellence
OIHP	Office International D'Hygiene Publique

Public Health

Chapter 1
What is public health?

Public health is a term much used in the media, and by health professionals and activists. They speak of a 'public health approach' or a 'public health policy' for a particular health issue. Governments organize themselves with ministries or departments of public health at the national or the local level. International agencies such as the World Health Organization (WHO) promote public health policies and regional organizations such as the European Union also have their public health funding and policies. But what does all this mean? What do these agencies and institutions see as the area of action under this broad heading?

Everyone knows what a health service is, but ideas about what public health is are more blurred. The public is confused about public health and uncertain what it means in practice. In the UK they might associate public health with cleanliness or with sanitation, with environmental health and inspections of housing or of food outlets. Professionals working in the public health field would see it differently—but they would not agree among themselves either. They might see it as something called 'health promotion' or as activities called 'social marketing'. In the United States or in Southern or Northern Europe, the focus would be different. The public health traditions in these countries vary in line with their different histories. For example, in the United States litigation on public health issues is common, but state involvement is less so, while some Scandinavian countries have a tradition of state involvement or even state ownership of industries such as alcohol which are connected with public health.

Public health is contested and without a single agreed definition. One recent text referred to the 'amoeba-like nature' of public health. A classic definition comes from nearly a century ago, from the American public health expert C. E. A. Winslow:

> Public health is the science and art of preventing disease, prolonging life and promoting physical health and efficiency through organized community efforts for the sanitation of the environment, the control of community infections, the education of the individual in principles of personal hygiene, the organisation of medical and nursing services for the early diagnosis and preventive treatment of disease, and the development of social machinery which will ensure to every individual in the community a standard of living adequate for the maintenance of health.

Nearly seventy years ago in 1948, the WHO defined health as 'a state of complete physical, mental and social wellbeing and not merely the absence of disease or infirmity'. This was a very wide-ranging definition, which also gives an idea of the breadth of the public health agenda.

Public health is a very broad concept. In its narrowest sense, it refers to the health of a population, the longevity of individual members, and their freedom from disease. But it can also be anticipatory, geared to the prevention of illness rather than simply the provision of care and treatment. It is concerned with the promotion of health and well-being in its widest sense, the wider determinants of health and a general sense of common interest or good. It can be concerned with identifying longer term risks to health and trends rather than immediate threats which require medical intervention. It deals with healthy as well as sick people and is a separate concept from health services, which deal with the sick population.

Public health can therefore lack coherence. Different interests have different conceptions of public health and define it according to political and other concerns. These definitions connect with ideas about the role of the state and the protection of individual liberty. Strategies and policies will be shaped by the interplay with government and wider forces in society.

Time also alters public health. Definitions of public health are not the same over time. Two recent examples of this tell us something about why this happens.

In 1988, a report on the public health function produced by Sir Donald Acheson, then the British Chief Medical Officer, the central government public health official, described public health as 'the science and art of preventing disease, prolonging life, and promoting health through the organised efforts of society'.

Sixteen years later, a British businessman, Derek Wanless, was commissioned by the Treasury, the government finance department, to review public health policy and practice. His definition of public health drew on Acheson's but was significantly different. In 2004 it was:

> The science and art of preventing disease, prolonging life and promoting health through the organised efforts *and informed choices* of society, *organisations, public and private, communities and individuals.*

The change in definitions and their origin is instructive. In 1988, a public health doctor working in a health ministry produced the definition. Nearly two decades later, a businessman working for the finance ministry was the agent of public health. This tells us something about the politics of public health at those points in time. And so too does the change in definitions. Those involved in the later formulation of public health now included the private as well as the public sector but also a range of voluntary organizations, and there was a strong role for individual responsibility through informed choice. Wanless wanted what he called a 'fully engaged' scenario, where individuals took responsibility for their health and health services were responsive to their needs. The changed definition and the ministry which produced it reflected the politics of the early 21st century, just as Acheson's earlier formulation was an outgrowth of the late 1980s and the revival of public health in the wake of HIV/AIDS. This was nothing new for public health for it has always been the outgrowth of the forces and the interests operational at the time.

Change over time is the key to understanding public health. This book draws attention to the very earliest history of public health 4,000 years ago. A modern history of public health then began in the 18th century with efforts by governments to deal with environmental problems. An emphasis on the environment and on sanitation was the key to public health in the 18th and for much of the 19th centuries. Rapid economic growth and mass urbanization coincided with high mortality from infectious diseases such as cholera and typhus.

In the latter half of the 19th century came a change. From the 1860s, when Louis Pasteur formulated germ theory, bacteriology opened up a different view of public health with the possibility of vaccines and therapies for specific diseases, with safe food and water and infant feeding practices also coming on to the agenda. The focus of public health began to shift from collective management of the environment to interventions targeted at the individual in the home.

A further stage emerged by the mid-20th century, as this version of public health began to seem less relevant when access to health services, however funded, was more widespread. The old killer diseases such as tuberculosis were in decline. The arrival of welfare states gave greater security and also access to public housing. Public health went through a period of reorientation and came to focus on diseases of lifestyle, including various cancers and cardiovascular disease. Individual lifestyle and its modification became a key element in public health.

Then from the 1980s came further change. The arrival of HIV/AIDS was a reminder that the risk of infectious disease was still present, even in Western societies. Evidence of the health risks of climate change brought the environment back on to the public health agenda. One can think of stages of public health, from the 19th-century concern with the environment to the present day, when public health can be a matter of genetics and ethics. The language which has been used to define public health illustrates these changing scenarios: terms used in the UK since the 19th century have included public health; hygiene(including social hygiene and racial hygiene); community medicine; social medicine; public health medicine; and then public health again more recently.

How to segment public health?

Many attempts have been made to organize the different components of public health within a coherent framework. In 2005, the UK Faculty of Public Health, the national public health professional body, attempted this task and grouped what was called the 'public health function' into three areas or domains. These were:

> *Health improvement*, which meant promoting healthy lifestyles and healthy environments and encompassing issues of inequality and the wider social determinants of health.
>
> *Health protection*, which meant protecting people from specific threats to their health, including such activities as

immunization and vaccination, screening, injury prevention, control of infectious diseases, and emergency planning.

Health service improvement, which meant bringing an evidence-based population perspective to planning, commissioning, and evaluating services and interventions to ensure they are effective, high quality, safe, and supporting clinical governance.

The faculty's definition tended to be health service focused because this was where the public health profession was located at that time. Later, formal public health services in the UK moved into local government and so there were efforts to modify this framework to account for changed circumstances. A Public Health Outcomes Framework built on the earlier segmentation but placed stronger emphasis on the reduction of health inequalities. Such changes underline the constantly shifting focus of public health.

There have been attempts to represent public health and the influences on it in visual terms. The 'rainbow diagram' produced by public health academics Dahlgren and Whitehead in the early 1990s illustrated the complex interaction of social factors and the range of sectors across which actions would need to be taken to influence the health of populations (Figure 1).

After Dahlgren and Whitehead produced their diagram (which altered even between 1991 and 1992, substituting 'hereditary factors' for 'constitutional factors' as one influence) discussion of public health changed again. There was a growing recognition of the global dimension of public health and the threats posed by bioterrorism, climate change, and by outbreaks of infectious disease with the potential to become pandemics. A revised version of the rainbow diagram published in 2006 reflected this (Figure 2).

A more pragmatic way of understanding public health is to think of it in its various manifestations, in an *institutional* or state

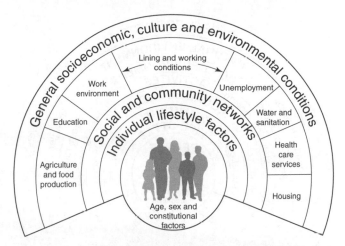

1. **The Dahlgren and Whitehead 'rainbow diagram', representing the interaction of social factors and the range of sectors where action needs to be taken to influence public health.**

administration context; as a *profession*; and also as a form of *knowledge* or *ideology*, with research and science increasingly playing its part.

We might, in this context, think of who is likely to be involved in public health and their location. In the UK, for example, this could currently be the Chief Medical Officer in the Department of Health; a director of public health in local government; an employee in the national agency, Public Health England, or maybe NICE (National Institute for Health and Care Excellence), whose role is to assess the evidence on public health interventions; someone involved in a health activist group such as ASH (Action on Smoking and Health); or a public health academic, maybe an epidemiologist or a policy analyst working in a university. In other countries, the personnel and organizations would be different. Not all countries have central officials or agencies dealing with public health, and sometimes, as in Australia in recent history, they come and go because of politics. A central public health agency was

7

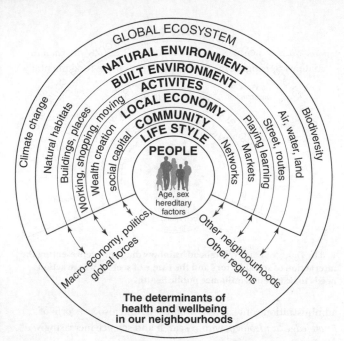

GLOBAL ECOSYSTEM

NATURAL ENVIRONMENT

BUILT ENVIRONMENT

ACTIVITES

LOCAL ECONOMY

COMMUNITY

LIFE STYLE

PEOPLE

Age, sex
hereditary
factors

Climate change

Natural habitats

Buildings, places

Working, shopping, moving

Wealth creation

social capital

Networks

Markets

Street, routes

Playing learning

Air, water, land

Biodiversity

Macro-economy, politics,
global forces

Other neighbourhoods
Other regions

**The determinants of
health and wellbeing
in our neighbourhoods**

2. **Public health changes over time—this later version of the 'rainbow diagram' represents a recognition of the global dimensions of public health which have appeared on the agenda in recent decades.**

established there under a Labour government but did not survive a subsequent change in government.

Critiques of public health

The lack of a clear definition for public health has led to criticism. What is meant by 'health', or by 'the public' and by 'public health', can be subject to endless debate and redefinition. Here is an introduction to some ongoing arguments which affect public health.

Should public health focus on achievable technical solutions or aim at wider social change? Public health has been criticized for

8

preferring 'technical fixes', short-term interventions which help deal with a particular issue, to fundamental reappraisals of society. It is easier to develop vaccination programmes than to initiate wide-ranging measures which deal more fundamentally with poverty and social inequality and consequently to better health for poorer classes. This critique draws attention to the potential political role of public health, which some argue should be at the core of what it does.

Does public health entail a 'nanny state'? Another area of fundamental debate has been the tension between the collective benefits to society of public health interventions contrasted with the liberty of individuals. It is seen as unfair for the majority of individuals to sacrifice their individual freedom for a common good which may be illusory. This was a key area of debate during the early public health reforms in the 19th century, and resurfaced in a different form with discussions of the 'nanny state' in more recent times. In this recent debate it was argued that it was not the role of government to lecture populations about habits which only affected individuals or which might not lead to ill health for many years. It was the individual's choice about how he or she lived their lives. This critique has also surfaced in public responses to vaccination, a long-standing arena of public health dissent. The population good conferred by vaccination contrasts with the individual damage it might cause.

Do professional interests define public health? Because public health has lacked an agreed definition, it has been argued that public health professionals have defined the tasks which they undertake as being public health, without a clear rationale for what that means. So what is 'public health' has been dependent on the positioning of the profession at particular points in time. For example 'public health' only took an interest in health inequality in the UK in the early 1980s when the professional position of public health doctors in health services had been undermined by structural changes. In the 1930s it ran an extensive network of health services and became preoccupied with administration rather than action in local communities. Whether public health is a medical or non-medical profession is also important and this varies between countries.

Does economic development achieve more than public health interventions? A long-standing debate in the field raises the question of the benefits of formal public health intervention versus more general economic improvement. This debate started with the social medicine academic Thomas McKeown in the 1970s. He argued, using historical data, that formal public health interventions achieved less than more general economic improvement secured through raised standards of living and better nutrition. The political issue was whether state intervention achieved more than economic growth and the role of the market, which might bring improvements in population health in their train.

Is public health a form of surveillance of society and medicalization? The critique advanced by the French philosopher Michel Foucault has been influential in academic circles. It saw public health as part of the 'medicalization' of society from the 18th century and the extension of state power. Public health, in this interpretation, has the role of surveillance of the poor in the interests of the ruling and middle classes of society. Public health techniques such as screening or the health survey have their role in state surveillance. They medicalize areas of life only indirectly connected with disease.

Many such commentaries are implicitly critical of public health and its aims. They contrast with the social purpose, enthusiasm, and activism which characterizes the public health field. Let us now turn to look at some challenges facing this very broad field.

Chapter 2
Current challenges

What is the overall context within which public health is operating? What has been happening to the health of the public? Public health is at a substantial crossroads. Most populations worldwide have seen gains in life expectancy over the last half century. Fertility rates have been declining. The profile of major causes of disease and death has been changing; in low and middle income countries non-communicable diseases are replacing previously dominant infectious diseases. In many countries there has been a rise in overweight people and obesity. The pattern of infectious diseases is changing, with an increased rate of emergence of new infectious diseases and a widespread increase in antibiotic resistance. Increased globalization of trade and industry, the movement of populations, and global environmental conditions are changing in response to the widespread pressures of economic activity. Public health thus faces many challenges.

Public health operates at different levels: global, national, and local. This chapter looks first at the national and local levels, taking the UK as the main example with some cross-national comparison. In 2014, the UK Faculty of Public Health, the professional organization for public health, reported a members' survey about the priorities for the coming year. These were:

- minimum unit pricing for alcohol
- standard tobacco packaging
- reduction of personal transport use
- the living wage
- physical activity targets reinstated by government
- 20 per cent duty on alcoholic beverages
- reformulation of food products to cut sugar
- ending the marketing of high fat and sugar products to children
- excluding the NHS from US and EU trade agreements which might affect the ability to take back contracted-out services into the public sector
- reinstating the Secretary of State for Health's responsibility for the NHS
- a 20 mph limit in built up areas
- to have personal and social health education as a statutory duty in all schools.

Not in the top twelve, but with strong support were: antimicrobial resistance; climate change; inequality with a particular emphasis on young people; and 'systems issues'.

Such a listing gives a sense of the range of public health interests, and not just in the UK—there are *topics* such as smoking, alcohol consumption, physical activity, the health effects of transport, food and diet; *public health strategies* such as health education; a concern for formal *health services*, in this case the NHS; a focus on *target groups and age ranges*, young people in this instance; and also *cross-cutting macro-issues* such as climate change and inequality. Some topics were long-standing and others relatively new.

The annual report of the British Chief Medical Officer (CMO), the leading public health official in government, for the ten years 2004–14 gave a similar range of concerns. In 2004, the topics were second-hand smoke and smoke-free public areas; obesity; MRSA infection in hospitals; tuberculosis and its rise; cross-border cigarette smuggling; HIV prevention; and chronic obstructive pulmonary disease. In 2011, under a new CMO, Dame Sally Davies, the focus was liver disease and its rise—related to obesity, undiagnosed hepatitis, and alcohol consumption; diabetes and access to health care; mental health; and well-being.

The WHO produced a national burden of disease toolkit where risk factors were based on lifestyle, and medical and environmental factors—tobacco, alcohol, blood pressure, high cholesterol, the consumption of fruit and vegetables, occupational health, and sexual health. To this the CMO added urban outdoor air pollution; social determinants of health (based on a review conducted by the epidemiologist Sir Michael Marmot), with issues of the early years of life; cognitive issues and education; employment; standard of living; and the role of communities.

These listings—and their change over time—give a sense of the almost impossibly broad agenda of public health. But a pattern was discernible which was congruent with the listing from the Faculty of Public Health—there were some key topics, changing over time; a focus on particular groups, again young or very young people were prominent; the relationship with formal health services; and strategies which varied from those focused on the individual to a more general concern to change the environment or social and economic circumstances.

In order to bring some order to this cacophony, we will examine the current range of public health activities segmented in the way we discussed in Chapter 1—first, current central topics which illustrate the *ideology* of public health and the *tactics* used, then the *personnel and professions* involved and the *institutional/state locations*. First the local and national level is covered and then the global/international sphere.

The ideology of public health: topics and tactics

Many of the topics with which public health in concerned relate to a concern for what is termed *lifestyle and its modification*. Smoking was a key example of this, and the 2004 English legislation on smoke-free areas, stimulated in part by developments in Ireland and Scotland, was seen as a great step forward in terms of making smoking culturally unacceptable, moves which had taken place earlier in cities such as New York. Smoking remained a central campaigning issue for public health. Legislation on plain packaging had been introduced in countries such as Australia and was planned in the UK, and cross-border smuggling of cigarettes was still a concern.

The advent of electronic cigarettes in the early 21st century and support from consumers brought dilemmas for the public health field nationally and internationally. Were they an innovation to be welcomed, providing a less harmful way to smoke and a potential route out of smoking, or were they a 'Trojan horse' with tobacco industry support designed to 'renormalize' smoking? Smoking had long been an area where cultural issues were a central battleground. Again there were cross-national differences. In Australia e-cigarettes were banned and there was no national debate, while in the UK a vigorous debate in the public health field built on traditions of nicotine harm reduction in scientific circles. In the US there was a proposal for modest regulation at Federal level but some states had applied tobacco regulation to e-cigarettes.

Alcohol was another lifestyle issue with widespread concern about 'binge drinking', about youth drinking, in particular that of young women, and with a move to win acceptance of the public health tactic of minimum unit pricing. The UK had introduced longer drinking hours in the early 21st century, in Australia drinking hours had been restricted, while in the US the legal drinking age was, at 21, much higher. The aim in the UK and elsewhere was to change a general culture where drinking was considered acceptable as a regular daily activity and where there were steep rises in liver disease.

But there were countervailing trends, including the rise in non-drinking young people. Dismissed by some commentators as merely a reflection of Britain's multi-ethnic community and the Muslim presence, this trend had nevertheless been apparent for some time. In 2013, one in five adults were teetotal and the proportion of young people (16–24) who were non-drinkers had increased 40 per cent between 2005 and 2013. Concern shifted to older people's drinking. There were significant national differences even within the UK, with Scotland playing a leading role in attempts to initiate measures like minimum unit pricing. In countries like Australia that tactic was not important, while the US had more stringent restrictions and a society where social controls on drinking were generally stronger.

The obesity 'epidemic' moved centre stage with a major report from a government enquiry, Foresight, published in 2007. Government modelling estimated that, by 2050, 60 per cent of adult men, 50 per cent of adult women, and about 25 per cent of all children under 16 could be obese. Diet and physical activity—changes in personal lifestyle—were seen as part of the solution. But there was also increasing emphasis on more technical responses: the role of bariatric surgery as a 'magic bullet'.

Sexual health too remained on the agenda, no longer just HIV/AIDS as was the case in the 1980s, but a general concern about the rise in sexually transmitted diseases (STDs), and the poor sexual health of young people. The rate of teenage conceptions, which had caused concern, was falling, for example a decrease of 10 per cent in women under 18 between 2011 and 2012. Mortality from traditional public health concerns such as heart disease was in decline, but with clear social class differences.

Other public health topics were more recent arrivals on the agenda, even if they reformulated past concerns. Mental health was an earlier concern for public health. In recent years, it re-emerged as a public health topic, with dementia at one end of the lifecycle but also depression and suicide among younger men. Relationships developed between public health and psychiatric interests. The rise in hospital infections and MRSA led to a revival of focus on handwashing, basic cleanliness, and the control of infection.

Infectious disease was no longer the central public health issue in the UK or other developed countries that it had been in the past. But it had grown in importance, and the role of pandemic planning for swine and bird flu was an important aspect of public health work in the 21st century. Action against external threat of infection was a strand of public health work called health protection. In the 21st century, this took on a new dimension as new external threats appeared. The threat of bioterrorism, the spread of deadly disease by dissident political groups, caused concern. In 2006, the assassination of the Russian dissident Alexander Litvinenko by the use of the radioactive drug polonium in central London led to a major public health scare. Food safety and security was also high profile. The internationalization of the food trade was behind public health scandals, for example the unauthorized use of horsemeat by suppliers of supermarkets which came to light in 2013.

The *tactics* employed by public health were varied, and embedded in a variety of locations. *Vaccination* was an important, long-standing, and controversial strategy. Nearly all children were immunized against tetanus, diphtheria, whooping cough, *Haemophilus influenzae* b, meningitis C, and measles, mumps, and rubella (MMR). The combined MMR vaccine was introduced in 1988, but questions over its safety led to widespread concerns on the part of parents and the media, and to an initial fall in those being immunized to below 80 per cent in 2003–4. The decline in trust was blamed on research which was later proved to be faulty and which linked the vaccine to autism. This decline in coverage also reflected long-standing public fears about vaccination. Vaccination as a mode of prevention of cervical cancer was introduced for teenage girls in 2008 initially for 11–12 and 17–18 year olds, and since 2014 was routinely recommended at ages 12–14. This was, perhaps surprisingly, much less controversial than vaccination in other areas. Other countries had more stringent regulations around vaccination—for example in Australia and the US, vaccination certificates were needed for children starting school.

Screening as a mode of prevention came into the public health field when tuberculosis was widespread, and mass screening of civilians for the disease began in the UK in 1945. Screening for cervical cancer and breast cancer was established, in the latter case from the 1980s. More recently, screening for bowel cancer and prostate cancer has been introduced. Such techniques were criticized because they raised the possibility of overdiagnosis and unnecessary treatment of conditions which might never progress; the advice given by the National Screening Service on breast cancer screening was modified to reflect the uncertainty in this area. Age discrimination became an issue, with screening not automatically available for those over 70, the ages when a higher proportion of cancers occurred.

Screening was carried out in a hospital or in a general practitioner's (GP's) surgery, and the history of how different screening services came to be located in different settings indicated the tensions between different professional and service interests involved. It was a procedure allied to health services, although sometimes based in the hospital and sometimes in primary care.

Another major recent development—*medication as prevention*—also demonstrated a public health initiative operating in a health service setting. Taking medicines on a long-term basis to prevent disease developing, as a mode of maintaining good health, was widespread. The sharp rise in the use of statins to reduce cholesterol and thus the rate of heart disease was a key initiative which developed from the late 20th century. British Heart Foundation figures published in 2011 showed annual statin prescriptions in England soared from 295,000 to 52 million between 1981 and 2008. Prescriptions for lipid-lowering drugs trebled between 2003 and 2013. There were other examples of prescription as public health prevention—the prescription of methadone to drug users on a long-term basis became common from the 1990s, and nicotine replacement therapy was also used as a smoking prevention strategy. More recently pre-exposure prophylaxis for HIV prevention has started in low income countries (LICs) and is due to expand. This focus on medication brought public health into a closer relationship with the pharmaceutical industry.

Medication was far from the traditional public health strategy of *health education, information, and persuasion.* That tactic still continued although with significant changes. The national health education function no longer existed in the UK by the late 20th century, and public health campaigns were promoted by a variety of different agencies, including, in the alcohol field, Drinkaware, funded by the alcohol industry. A general public health campaign, Change4Life, had run for a number of years and recommendations were tied to best practice as identified by the government agency NICE, which took on public health as part of its quality standards work in 2013.

In the 1960s and 1970s, campaigns had been directed at the whole population and this continued with the AIDS campaigns of the 1980s. But changes in media technology meant that there was a move towards using social media to reach young people, so that the public health message could be segmented, tailored, and targeted. This strategy mirrored the changes in the way in which the industries producing products like alcohol and food were also reaching out to their consumers.

Health education and the way information was presented also changed in other ways. Food labelling was one initiative, and there was controversy about whether a government or industry-sponsored scheme should be adopted. The post-2010 coalition government in the UK began to talk about what it called 'nudge'—tactics which might move individuals towards more healthy behaviours. A new public health approach called 'behavioural economics' lay behind the use of strategies such as payment by results. Would individuals behave more healthily if they were given financial incentives? Why people made the choices they did became the subject of 'anthropology of choice'. David Hunter, a public health academic, wrote of the tensions between the 'nudge' and 'shove' approaches in public health (the smoking ban was an example of the latter).

The links with industry in the public health field were controversial. *Partnership* in general was a key issue, at the local level, where loose alliances of different interests coalesced around different public health issues. Alcohol had been one example, potentially bringing together the voluntary sector, licensing, alcohol treatment interests, the retail sector, and others. At the national level, the issue was whether industry interests should be party to such alliances. Historically, many in the public health field were hostile to cooperation. In the UK, the government's Responsibility Deal launched in 2011, which brought together public health personnel with industry interests for food and alcohol, was riven by dissent. However in other areas, for example prevention as medication, industry links with public health became closer, although in this case it was the pharmaceutical industry. The arrival of e-cigarettes, where some companies had been taken over by the tobacco industry, brought tensions to a head.

Public health people and professions

Which professions deliver public health is significant and changes from one country to another over time. Public health in the UK had been a medical occupation. By the late 1990s a move to change the professional focus of public health took root because the remit of public health was so wide that it could not be encompassed simply by medically qualified personnel. Multidisciplinary public health came on to the agenda. In 2000, the Faculty of Public Health dropped the suffix 'Medicine' in its title and opened membership to non-medically qualified people bringing expertise from backgrounds in the social sciences, geography, politics, economics, health intelligence, and other areas (including history). Common training requirements were developed, posts opened up to both medical and non-medical entrants, and a form of regulation for non-medical specialists was established. In a report in 2001 the CMO identified three levels of the public health workforce: specialist, practitioner, and the wider workforce.

The practitioner workforce involved a wide range of occupations—from health visitors and community nurses to health promotion practitioners and environmental health officers, and occupational health and trading standards staff. Their day-to-day responsibility was to influence population health, although some would have obtained their training in other areas such as teaching or clinical practice. The most diverse area was the wider workforce, which included people at all levels and in all sectors. These included journalists, pharmacists, social care staff, teachers, workers in the retail or hospitality sectors, town planners, and those working on the built environment. Both actually and potentially there was a vast army of public health workers.

This style of workforce was specific to the UK and in other countries the pattern of the workforce was different. In the United States, public health historically had been far less medically dominated than in the UK. In Australia, public health as a profession was weaker with fewer public health posts in health systems.

NGOs (non-governmental organizations) or voluntary groups in the public health arena were also an important force. Activist 'single issue' groups operated to raise awareness of particular issues. In recent years the Alcohol Health Alliance in the UK showed how to promote a public health issue. Led by the President of the Royal College of Physicians, Sir Ian Gilmour, the alliance brought together a range of different scientific and clinical disciplines with public health personnel concerned about rising levels of alcohol consumption and harm. It made its case through the media and through policy advocacy. Other countries also had advocacy bodies, for example the American Public Health Association or the Cancer Councils in Australia, which, building on the model of earlier AIDS councils, supported both research and advocacy.

Institutions and location

The institutional location of public health was important. Public health can operate in different ways at national and local levels. In the US, there was the Surgeon General at the national level and also state public health departments. American public health tended to focus only on the poor, with other prevention services available on a paying basis. Much activity also took place through the medium of the law courts, and there was also the option of local state referenda, such as those which brought the legalization of medical cannabis in the 21st century in several US states.

In the UK in 2012, the Health and Social Care Act, part of the wide-ranging reorganization of health services under the coalition government, gave local authorities duties to improve the health of their local population and required them to appoint a director of public health. Public health moved out of health services and into local government, a move which was seen in some circles as 'coming home' because services were returning to where they had been positioned and funded both prior to the establishment of the NHS and up to the early 1970s. Different systems operated in different parts of the UK, with public health in Scotland operating in the health boards which all had large public health departments. Scotland, as we will see, had a distinctive public health history which enabled it to take the lead on public health issues sometimes earlier than, and then influencing, England.

Cross-cutting issues: inequalities

The single issue focus of public health has been criticized for failing to look at some of the wider determinants of health issues. Health inequalities and the social determinants of health came more centrally into health debates in the 21st century after a period in the 1980s and 1990s when it was not possible to raise the topic openly.

Visual representations of inequality highlighted the geographical variation in death rates. In London, life expectancy varied along the tube lines. In the London borough of Camden, residents of Hampstead in north-west London could expect to live longer than their counterparts in Somers Town in the south of the borough. Inequality 'slopes' were published for every local authority in the country, and gave a telling representation of the class and spatial nature of health inequality. Geographers showed that these patterns corresponded with those a century earlier, demonstrating the enduring nature of inequality.

The publication of Richard Wilkinson and Kate Pickett's book *The Spirit Level: Why Equality Is Better for Everyone* in 2010 engendered wide debate at both national and international levels about whether less equal societies were also less healthy. The WHO's Global Commission on the Social Determinants of Health was published in 2008. It said that empowerment had three dimensions: material (money, education, employment), psychosocial (having control over one's life), and political (having a voice). At the national level too, the social determinants of health—defined as early child development, education, and employment—were important in giving people control over their lives.

The focus on early years interventions, the first months and years of life, was characteristic of public health. Getting the start right and tackling intergenerational issues had long been a public health concern. Poor housing and diet, and unemployment, were transmitted from parent to child and 'breaking the cycle' was seen as a challenge. The focus, it was argued, should be the home or the school as well as the relationship to health services. This argument had strong historical resonance.

Public health was an international and a regional enterprise. The European Union had expanded its role in public health after the Maastricht Treaty of 1992, and European regulation was important in areas such as smoking and food safety. The health problems of Eastern Europe also came on to the agenda after the end of communism and the USSR. Disparities in health between East and West Germany and, outside the EU, Russian levels of alcohol consumption were only two of the issues. Migration also became a public health issue for the EU alongside the other issues which it raised for those countries. Public health had long been marked by the transfer of influences and initiatives from one country to another. The arrival of the EU on the public health scene added a new geographic dimension.

Canada, Australia, and New Zealand had influenced public health in Britain previously, and British influences had also been felt in those countries. Canada played a pioneering role in new public health approaches from the 1970s, as we will see in Chapter 6. Australia too developed pioneering approaches in smoking and HIV/AIDS prevention, as discussed in Chapter 5. This network of cross-national influences, also including the US, began in the post-World War II years and has continued to the present, augmented more recently by European public health activity.

Globalization and public health

A new terminology—that of globalization and global health governance—is now used within public health. Globalization is defined as a set of global processes which intensify the interconnected nature of human interaction across economic, political, cultural, and environmental spheres. Global health has expanded as a field of study, research, and action. International health was the earlier term used in the public health field. Global health is seen as different, involving a wide range of disciplines and policy actors beyond the state, including civil society organizations, and also relationships worldwide, not just between individual states.

New public health challenges resulted from the increase in human mobility, driven by factors such as the increase in air, sea, and land transport, the growth of tourism and business travel, conflicts and civil unrest, changes in the global economy, and greater liberalization of markets and migration policies. The rapid spread of SARS (Severe Acute Respiratory Syndrome) in 2003 exemplified the public health implications of these trends. The first case was identified in Guangdong province in China in February 2003, when an infected physician spent the night in a hotel in the Hong Kong district of Kowloon. By the end of February, the disease began spreading globally along air routes as guests at the same hotel flew home—to Canada, Singapore, and other countries. In August 2003, when the WHO declared the world SARS free, the disease had spread to twenty-nine countries, resulting in over 8,000 probable cases and 774 deaths worldwide. Air transport also played a key role in the global spread of influenza H1N1 (known as 'swine flu') with cases in at least 171 countries during the first months of the 2009 pandemic.

The 'Big Three'—the disease triumvirate of malaria, HIV/AIDS, and tuberculosis—dominated the interests of global health organizations and funders in the early 21st century. The abrupt transition to global capitalism in Russia after the end of the Soviet Union, and the resulting collapse of the health system, led to the explosion of tuberculosis there from the early 1990s, while incomplete drug courses received by many caused drug resistance. Malaria remained an important disease. Malaria transmission was determined by climate features and ecology, but inadequate access to prevention methods such as bed nets and repellents, weak health systems, lack of funding for government control programmes, and substandard housing enhanced the risk of infection. These issues came to the fore again in the discussion of responses to the Ebola epidemic in West Africa in 2014–15.

A range of international organizations dealt with these international or global public health issues. Some, such as WHO and UNICEF, had been involved since the 1940s, but their role had been contested in recent times. Other players such as the World Bank or the World Trade Organization (WTO) were more recent entrants to the global health scene. The role of the WTO was controversial in the protection and enforcement of trade-related intellectual property rights or TRIPS. When such rights were applied to the development of new drugs for tuberculosis or antiretroviral treatments for HIV/AIDS, controversy resulted and forced the WTO to acknowledge its role in responding to public health emergencies. The WTO acknowledged the right to health of all its member states in the 2001 Doha Declaration.

The private health foundations were new entrants to the global field, although with historic antecedents discussed in Chapter 6. The Bill and Melinda Gates Foundation concentrated on disease eradication through vaccination. In 2010, Gates provided 7 per cent of total development assistance for health. The foundation's key targets were malaria, guinea worm, HIV/AIDS, and polio.

Global public–private partnerships characterized a range of arrangements which came into global health from the late 1980s into the 21st century. These covered a diverse set of health issues such as HIV/AIDS, tuberculosis, malaria, vaccines, drugs for neglected tropical diseases, schistosomiasis, diarrhoea control, handwashing, and reproductive health. Some of the largest and best known included the Global Fund to Fight AIDS, Tuberculosis and Malaria, established in 2002 and with a board made up of donor countries, multilateral partners, and representatives of civil society and the private sector; the GAVI Alliance, set up in 2000; and the President's Emergency Fund for AIDS Relief. In some low and middle income countries, external funding for HIV/AIDS exceeded the internal funds available for health systems as a whole.

Commentators criticized the lack of legitimacy and transparency of the funds in relation to the people at whom they directed their efforts. They were answerable only to funders and their scope tended to be limited only to infectious diseases. Their existence in the public health field had brought with it a focus on measurable 'results', with neglect of areas where improvement was less easy to quantify, for example community home-based care. The foundations tended to focus on 'technical fixes' such as vaccination. Gates, for example, had invested massively in anti-polio strategies.

Globalization also affected tobacco and alcohol. The anti-tobacco movement had moved outside the developed world. It is estimated that by 2030 low and middle income countries would account for around 70 per cent of all tobacco-related deaths. In China, annual tobacco deaths were expected to reach two million by 2025. Transnational tobacco corporations developed worldwide interests as their traditional markets in North America and Western Europe were eroded by anti-tobacco initiatives and changes in smoking culture. In the 1980s, corporations asked the GATT (General Agreement on Tariffs and Trade), the predecessor to the WTO, to challenge government monopolies and to gain access to South East Asian markets. Health objectives and trade objectives collided. The alcohol industry also followed a similar path, with a challenge under EU trade law to minimum unit pricing.

The Framework Convention on Tobacco Control, passed by the WHO in 2003, was the organization's first attempt to exercise its constitutional authority to develop a global public health treaty. The text of the convention failed to include language that would clarify its status in relation to existing trade agreements and lacked binding obligations, although issue-specific protocols might be signed. The first of these, on illicit trade, was in play during 2014. The convention encouraged countries to work to a common model of action, for example to ban tobacco advertising, promotion, and sponsorship, to raise taxation, and to develop measures to combat smuggling. The convention was a unique effort to regulate the activities of transnational corporations. There was no equivalent for alcohol or for food regulation, although some public health interests urged that its model should be followed there too.

Tobacco and alcohol are relatively traditional public health issues. Newer issues have been raised by global environmental change. Global climate change is the best known of these problems, occurring due to the excessive emission of greenhouse gases into the lower atmosphere, especially the release of carbon dioxide from fossil fuel combustion. According to the World Resources Institute, total global emissions grew 12.7 per cent between 2000 and 2005. The human population is described as a 'global geo physical force' affecting the planet and its functioning in unprecedented ways. Direct health impacts include those related to exposure to extremes of temperature (hot or cold), increases in extreme weather events (floods, cyclones, storm surges, droughts), and increased production of certain air pollutants and allergens. Decreases in winter mortality due to milder weather might compensate for higher rates of summer deaths due to heatwaves. There is discussion about the need to achieve sustainable environmental and social conditions, maintaining the ecological systems and processes on which healthy life depends.

Security also came on to the global agenda in an era of wars, pestilence, and civil unrest. Health issues have been included in the traditional issues of national security and at the global level, for example in the 1997 Institute of Medicine's report for the US National Academy, *America's Vital Interests in Global Health*. The spectre of biological weapons represented the clearest link between health and national security policy. Agents such as anthrax, plague, and smallpox presented a transnational problem. The 9/11 terrorist attacks on the World Trade Center in 2001 were followed by anthrax attacks—five letters containing *Bacillus anthracis* were mailed to US government officials and media outlets. Twenty-two people developed anthrax and five died. The incident caused great disruption with office buildings and postal facilities closed, mail irradiated, and 33,000 people requiring prophylaxis. The events led to large-scale efforts and collaboration between the public health and security communities to enhance preparedness in the event of a terrorist biological attack.

Public health thus faced a daunting range of challenges at both national and international/global levels. These presented political choices and dilemmas. Public health strategies also developed to deal with these issues. There was a growing emphasis, starting from the 1970s, on 'science' and 'evidence' to help understand the issues and inform policy making in a 'rational' way. A sizeable public health research community developed in many countries separate from the professional workforce, although connected with it. Public health academics formed international networks, and disciplines such as epidemiology, statistics, and heath economics came to the fore as key public health sciences. The methodology of the randomized controlled trial (random assignment of patients to two or more groups to test a specific drug or treatment) became the public health 'gold standard'.

But science was also controversial. The science could be subject to challenge, for example over climate change. It was not value free. Some commentators disputed the utility of public health interventions, arguing that clinical medicine had more to offer than prevention and the 'nanny state'. They criticized the nature of public health evidence. In some instances, for example e-cigarettes and their effects, the evidence became a policy and scientific battleground.

Chapter 3
The origins of public health into the 1700s

This book started by stating that public health cannot be understood without a knowledge of its history. The earliest roots of public health and its development up to the 18th century start the examination. Going back centuries highlights clear continuities between public health responses in the deeper past and in more recent times. These centuries show the development of public health responses as part of the armoury of the modernizing state, in association with military and economic needs; punitive responses to epidemic disease including the practice of quarantine; the association between health and morality; and the beginnings of scientific enquiry into public health issues, specifically through the development of statistics.

Throughout history, considering major health problems has entailed examining the health of the population as well as that of the individual. Evidence of activity concerned with the health of the community has been found in the very earliest civilizations. An urban civilization in the north of India which operated 4,000 years ago gives evidence of public health provision for its inhabitants. Sites excavated at Mohenjo-daro in the Indus Valley, and at Harappa in the Punjab, show these Indian cities were consciously planned in rectangular blocks apparently in accordance with building laws. Bathrooms and drains were common. The streets were broad, paved, and drained by covered sewers. The problem of obtaining adequate supplies of drinking water had largely been solved by pre-Christian cultures. The Cretan-Mycenaean culture had large conduits, and in the palace of Knossos on Crete there were bathing facilities and also water flushing arrangements for the toilets.

Theories about the health of the public came initially from the corpus of work associated with Hippocrates, the Greek physician who has become the fount of wisdom for healers of many types. The historical Hippocrates lived on the island of Kos, off the coast of present-day Turkey, from c.460 BC to 370 BC. Whether he wrote all, or indeed any, of the works attributed to him is less clear. The 'Hippocratic' writings are about sixty in number and they cover a wide range, from diagnostics to disease prevention. The great advantage of the range of the Hippocratic canon or corpus of work is its holistic nature. This has made Hippocrates attractive to modern medicine—the approach is always the whole patient. Hippocratic writings have been called the foundation of modern primary care. These writings talked about the four humours which were constitutive of health and disease. They were blood, yellow bile, black bile, and phlegm and were publicized by Galen, another giant of Greek medicine (129 AD–c.210 AD), who gave humoral medicine such prestige that it endured in medical thinking until the 18th century.

The Hippocratics viewed health as the result of a sound balance of the humours; humoral therapy was mixed, including diet, exercise, massage, and other interventions aimed at the individual patient. In some ways these conform to ideas of healthy living and lifestyle which have become common in more recent versions of public health. But there was also a different type of public health in the Hippocratic writings, because they were also aware that disease often swept through a community. In two well-known books, one on *Epidemics* and the other on *Airs, Waters, Places*, the Hippocratic writers reflected on these wider aspects of disease. The latter book was the first known attempt to relate environmental factors to disease and health, the foundation text of Western environmentalism. The writer distinguished between diseases which were always present in a population—*endemic*—and those which were not always present but sometimes became excessively frequent, or *epidemic*. Factors underpinning local endemicity were climate, soil, water, mode of life, and nutrition. The book reflected attempts to relate ideas about disease causation and prevention to specific social and economic circumstances. The seafaring Greeks needed to understand such relationships in order to select the best and healthiest sites for the establishment of new colonies.

The Romans also produced public health knowledge and practices which were compatible with their social and military organization. They were very successful as engineers and administrators, although dependent on the Greeks for much of their medical knowledge. Their aqueducts, bringing water to the cities, were a marvel of the ancient world. Roman public baths made personal hygiene and cleanliness possible for all citizens, and Roman administrative efficiency was deployed to develop public health services, public hospitals, and the employment of city physicians. The Romans were especially concerned with the bad effects of swampy grounds and marshy air. The poet, Marcus Terentius Varro, noted in 36 BC that tiny creatures bred in these places which were invisible to the naked eye but which entered the mouth and nose and caused disease.

Greek and Roman learning was transmitted by Arab scholars. Medieval Islamic medicine had a learned medical culture of its own and reformulated Greek ideas, adding new observations, medicines, and procedures. By the 10th century the majority of Greek medical works had been translated into Syriac, Hebrew, or Arabic. Cities had emptied out after the disintegration of the Roman empire in the west. But in the Middle Ages, urbanization gathered pace. Feudalism began to give way to new economic relationships based on free exchange: the trading societies of the late medieval world encouraged the growth of towns and cities. Health problems were dealt with initially in magical and religious terms. Disease was a punishment for sin and so prayer, penitence, and invocation of the saints were means employed to deal with health problems. But the body was the vessel of the soul so it was also important to strengthen it against the incursions of disease. Hence, as the public health historian George Rosen remarked, there was room for hygiene and public health in the Middle Ages.

As urban development expanded there was less preoccupation with the health of elites and more concern for the diseases of denser populations. The welfare of the needy was taken up by secular philanthropists with the approval of the Church, which had founded most of the initial hospitals. Hospitals were also established by knightly orders along their routes to the Crusades, including those of the Knights of St John, the Order of Hospitallers, who set up hospitals from Malta to Germany. The diseases of this far distant world are difficult to determine but evidence points towards the prevalence of smallpox, typhoid, diphtheria, cholera, typhus, anthrax, scarlet fever, measles, epilepsy, trachoma, and gonorrhoea. Malaria was also a prominent disease.

New diseases came to the fore as new methods of agricultural production developed in northern Europe from the early Middle Ages. The population of Europe is believed to have grown threefold between 800 and 1300. Increased agricultural production supported this expansion, but strained resources. Diseases of dietary deficiency expanded throughout the Middle Ages for the poor peasantry, who were often hungry. Population life expectancy at birth remained at 35 years. The average was influenced and much reduced by high infant and child mortality, and many people lived well beyond 35. It is estimated that 5 per cent lived beyond 60 even in ancient Rome. Malnutrition and undernutrition exacerbated the spread of diseases such as rickets, scurvy, and pellagra. One disease directly produced by crop failure was ergotism, or St Anthony's Fire, which resulted when whole communities consumed rye infected by the ergot fungus. Epidemic waves of this disease occurred from the 9th century.

Agricultural production changed, and so too did trading patterns between Europe and the urbanized societies of the Middle East. There were new opportunities for the spread of infections, plague, leprosy, tuberculosis, and the 'English sweats', now widely accepted to have been influenza. Tuberculosis increased alongside urbanization between 1000 and 1348. Tuberculosis of the lymph nodes in the neck became known as 'the king's evil' or 'the royal disease', and it was the custom for English and French kings to cure it by touching its victims. Exposure to tuberculosis confers immunity against leprosy and may be one reason for the decline in that disease in the late medieval period.

But it was leprosy and bubonic plague which caused some of the greatest suffering in the medieval period. Leprosy, relatively uncommon in the ancient world, had begun to spread in Europe early in the Middle Ages. It reached a terrifying peak during the 13th and 14th centuries, possibly expanding because it was associated with the large shifts of population produced by the Crusades. It gradually subsided after the 14th century; many lepers died as a result of the Black Death but also because of the association with tuberculosis. But it was not until the 16th century that leprosy lost all practical significance in Europe. Quarantine, the isolation of persons with infectious diseases, is a public health tactic which is still with us, most recently in the treatment of Ebola in West Africa and the isolation of people returning to England and the United States who have been infected.

Quarantine was used to deal with leprosy in medieval times. Then the Church, following precepts laid down in the book of Leviticus in the Old Testament, which associated spiritual with bodily uncleanliness, took the lead in the isolation of lepers. The diagnosis was often applied to a disease which might now be given another name. But it carried with it social ostracism and legal death. It condemned its victim to a life of isolation and begging, generally confined to a 'lazaretto', called after Lazarus, the poor man whose sores the dogs licked in Jesus' parable in the gospel of St Luke. Lepers needed to carry the leper's rattle when going outside so that passers by were alerted to the coming source of physical and moral contagion. Excommunication from the community was also motivated by the reputation of leprosy as a punishment for lechery and other sins; the disease may in fact have been confused with syphilis along with other skin conditions.

Epidemic bubonic plague produced a new relationship between disease and social disorder in late medieval Europe. It also stimulated the earliest direct involvement of civil government in the control and prevention of epidemic disease. The Black Death, starting in the late 1340s, was the first pandemic in history, a worldwide epidemic. It took more than four years to make its way via the Silk Road from the steppes of Central Asia to Western Europe, the Middle East, and North Africa. It decimated the population of Europe—between one-quarter and one-half are estimated to have died—and was the first of a series of epidemics which lost their hold only in the 1660s. Recently it has been asserted that the Black Death was not caused by the plague bacillus, *Yersinia pestis*, identified in Hong Kong by Alexandre Yersin in 1894. Various other organisms have been suggested since the Black Death did not conform completely to what is now known about the epidemiology of modern bubonic plague. Its rate of spread, seasonality, and mortality patterns, together with the fact that nobody noticed a lot of dead rats, have led some commentators to propose that anthrax, an unknown virus, or another infectious agent was the cause. Ergot poisoning has also been suggested, and even recently that the rats were in fact gerbils.

The problem, according to Bynum, is that these alternative interpretations concentrate almost entirely on the Black Death. In the plague years overall, from 1345 to 1666, the pattern is more certain. The collective historical experience, found in accounts of doctors and of those who had lived through more than one episode, was of a single repeated disease, almost certainly caused by the plague bacillus.

Health and morality had been connected in the response to leprosy, and morality was also seen as implicated in the Black Death. The range of explanations put forward at the time ranged from the wrath of God to sinfulness and sloth, the connection with marginal groups such as Jews or witches, and 'bad air'. Astrological causes were also frequently invoked. Plague stimulated forms of Christian penance such as the cult of public flagellation. But the frequent epidemics also drew forth measures of communal protection. Isolation, border controls, and compulsory confinement in hospital were combined with more general measures such as quarantine for ships coming from plague areas, control of the movement of persons and goods, and medical inspection. Italian port authorities began to turn away vessels travelling from suspect areas. In Venice in 1348, this action was formally codified, initially for a period of thirty days. Later this period was extended to forty days, hence the term 'quarantine'.

The development of Italian administrative measures to prevent the import and spread of plague in the 15th and 16th centuries subsequently provided a model which was copied by the rest of Europe. Permanent health boards began to be established in most major Italian cities during the early 16th century. Florence created one in 1527, followed by towns such as Pisa and Leghorn. In smaller towns, 'local gentlemen' were appointed as public health officers in time of epidemics. During epidemics, most health authorities had the power to isolate plague victims and their families and to destroy suspected goods and merchandise. Festivals, religious gatherings, and processions were banned in epidemic times despite the opposition of the clergy. The authority of the Church was challenged, and the Italian city health boards were admired and copied elsewhere in Europe.

England was relatively slow to follow, but controls were instituted under the Tudors and codified in a Plague Act of 1604. Its most important clause was to shut up the houses of plague victims—to isolate them, together with their families, for six weeks. Watchmen enforced the order and officers supplied the household with food. The rationale for this house arrest coincided with the aims of the Poor Law and other measures to deal with disorder arising from want. Migration stimulated by hunger or by plague was seen by the state as a threat to social stability. Both this plague clause and the enforced local settlement which was part of the Elizabethan Poor Law kept communities in place at times of social and economic disruption. The disappearance of plague from Europe after the last epidemic in Marseille in 1720–2 resulted from a combination of causes. It has been argued that the *cordon sanitaire* along the southern and eastern edges of the Austro-Hungarian empire may have had some effect in limiting spread. Other draconian measures may only have served to increase mortality.

Fears of social disorder were also matched by the dread of moral corruption which could result from disease. The issue of what would now be called STDs raised this in acute form. In the late 15th century, the disease which came to be called the French disease or pox, *morbus gallicus*, was believed to be a new contagion. It appeared in Italy in 1495 following Charles VIII's campaign against the Spaniards for control of Naples. His army, consisting of mercenaries from Belgium, Germany, France, Italy, and Spain, was believed to have spread the disease. In a way which later became characteristic of responses to epidemics, it was seen as the disease of foreigners. The Italians called it the 'French sickness' and the French called it the 'Neapolitan sickness'. The official historian of the House of Burgundy, Sebastian Brant, who had authored the satirical fable *The Ship of Fools*, provided the first illustrated account, with wood engravings by Dürer, who showed the syphilitic as a French fop (Figure 3). *Morbus gallicus* was the common name and the term syphilis was rarely used,

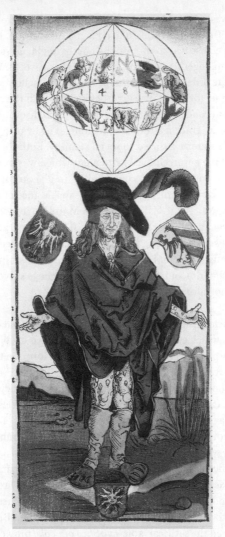

3. An early representation of a syphilitic by the German Albrecht
Dürer. It is true to type in representing him as a French 'fop'. Venereal
disease then, as later with HIV/AIDS, was seen within a moral
framework as a disease of 'the other'.

often referring to a range of conditions until the late 19th century when the specific bacterial origin of the disease was identified.

The disease's first appearance in Naples, where some of the Spanish mercenaries had been to the New World with Christopher Columbus, led to the assumption that this was a new disease imported from outside Europe. This 'Columbian exchange' is still debated by historians. The organism responsible for syphilis is *Treponema pallidum*, a spirochetal bacterium. The *Treponema* genus includes several species responsible for four different human diseases· pinta, yaws, endemic syphilis, and venereal syphilis. Historical epidemiologists have discounted the idea of the direct transmission of venereal syphilis from the Americas to Europe, although the transmission of a mutation of endemic syphilis is still considered a possibility. It was certainly considered a new disease in Europe at that time, and new measures to control its spread and that of the immorality it symbolized were put in place. France established stricter regulation and inspection of prostitutes from 1500. The arrival of *morbus gallicus* symbolized new attitudes towards the regulation of sexuality.

The 'Columbian exchange' worked in other ways. Military explorations, trade, and travel generated epidemics by exposing non-immune populations to new diseases. Smallpox, endemic in Europe, proved devastating to Native American populations in the New World. Europeans also brought malaria to the Americas. The internationalization of disease organisms through trade served to aid conquest. Such international factors have remained important in the transmission of disease and the public health response up to the present day—witness HIV/AIDS in recent times.

A new focus on science and investigation was associated with the rise of a new urban middle class whose wealth was dependent on commerce rather than on land. Their economic activities made possible the development of the national state, accompanied by a new secular culture. New approaches to the body emerged with close clinical observation giving descriptions of diseases such as whooping cough, typhus, and scarlet fever. Studies of disease transmission resulted in the first theory of contagious disease by Girolamo Fracastoro.

The growing interest in numerical calculations prompted the gathering of statistical information, initially in the Italian city states. Later, the development of what the French ideologue Condorcet called 'social mathematics' was significant in the relationship between the modern nation state and the health of its subjects. Methods for assessing the strength of the state by counting the population were developed by the late 17th-century physician, landowner, and social scientist, William Petty (1623–1687). He produced a 'political arithmetic of social facts' to enhance the state's chances of military defence, commercial and technological expansion, and social reform. He studied the conditions under which prosperity flourished and was impeded. Petty's friend, John Graunt (1620–1674), a mercer and fellow of the Royal Society, began to calculate statistics of health and disease. He looked at the London Bills of Mortality to discover the regularity of life events such as births and deaths, noting the excess of male over female births and excess male over female deaths. He also highlighted the higher urban than rural death rates.

The idea that the state required the development of statistics to define itself was primarily developed within the 18th-century German states, in particular Prussia. New theories of the state and the political and economic doctrines of mercantilism—the new system of trade and commerce—involved public health. These theories assumed that there was no distinction between the welfare of the state and the welfare of society. The interests of the state in building power and wealth required a large and healthy population. This approach supported public health in the authoritarian form of 'medical police'.

The best-known proponent of this approach was the Austrian physician, Johann Peter Franck (1745–1821), physician to the

18th-century Hapsburg court and director of the General Hospital in Vienna. In the multi-volume *System der vollstandigen medicinischen Polizey* (1779–1827), he outlined methods for regulating intimate individual behaviour which might spread or engender disease, such as marriage, pregnancy, and personal hygiene. He proposed public hygiene measures of drainage, pure water, and street cleaning. His system reflected the paternalistic political philosophy of 'cameralism' of the Hapsburg Empire, headed by enlightened despots who saw the role of the monarch as the parent of the people. The body and behaviour of the people was the property of the state, to be utilized for its benefit through the science of police, *policey*, a form of civil service administration. Franck's work was not simply that of a 'pioneer' of public health, but part of political struggles between an older concept of the authoritarian state and the more democratic ideals of the French Revolution. The French revolutionaries added health to the rights of man and asserted that health citizenship should be characteristic of the democratic state.

So by the 18th century, public health was becoming part of the modernizing state concerned with urbanization and economic development. In the century which followed its role was to become central to that state.

Chapter 4
Sanitation to education: 1800–1900s

A key period for public health came with the rise of the 'modern state' in the 19th century. Rapid economic growth and mass urbanization coincided with high mortality from infectious diseases such as cholera and typhus. Increases in life expectancy in the late 18th century juddered to a halt until the 1870s because of unhealthy urban environments. The definition and compass of public health at this time was about drains and sanitation, cleansing the environment as a whole. But this focus for public health changed during the century. Scientific breakthroughs in the 1860s, when the French chemist Louis Pasteur formulated germ theory, brought vaccines and pharmacotherapy for specific diseases. The environmental emphasis of 19th-century public health gave way to a greater focus on the individual, to education and personal advice, and to a concern for the health of mothers and babies in the home. This chapter will examine this period of challenge for public health and also the changing rationale of public health itself. The century was framed by issues which continue to mark public health.

Patterns of life expectancy

Britain was the world's first industrial nation and so initially the emphasis will be on what happened there.

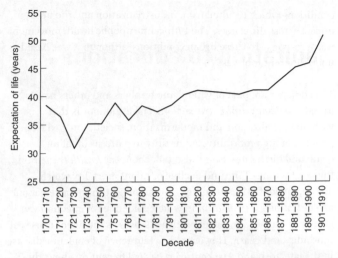

4. Life expectancy increased from the 18th to the early 20th century. But the plateau between the 1820s and the 1870s illustrates the human costs of industrialization and urbanization.

Figure 4 tells an overall story of an increase in life expectancy from the 18th century to the early 20th century. The average life expectancy at birth increased from around 31 years in the 1720s to about 50 years by the early 20th century, although approximately 10 per cent of the population lived beyond 60 in 18th-century France and Britain.

Oscillations in the 18th century have been related to changes in disease and in the food supply. But the most striking aspect of the graph is the plateau between the 1820s and the 1870s. Most of the increase in life expectancy occurred at the end of the 19th century. This pattern of life expectancy, when it stalled for such a long period, fuelled a long-standing debate among historians about the standard of living during the Industrial Revolution. Optimists about the effects of industrialization pointed to measurable improvements such as economic growth and rising incomes, while pessimists pointed to the poor living conditions which resulted from industrialization and the uneven impact across the classes. The 19th-century public health movement was a response to these urban conditions, although it was based upon different motives.

The statistics are part of what demographers and others have called the *demographic transition*. The argument is that with industrialization and modernization, societies moved from patterns of high mortality and fertility to patterns of falling death and birth rates. Some also talk about the *health transition*: the lengthening of life and decline of infant mortality which accompanied it. More recently, epidemiologists have talked about an *epidemiologic transition* in which epidemics of infection were gradually replaced by degenerative diseases as the major causes of morbidity and death. However, the resurgence of epidemic disease in the late 20th and 21st centuries has led to caution about this confident assertion.

Industrialization and urbanization

The debate was stimulated by the rapid pace of urbanization and population change in the 19th century (Figure 5). The population of Europe grew at a rapid rate, almost trebling between 1700 and 1890. The pace of change was fastest in England, and this and the rate of industrialization led to its characterization as the world's first industrial nation. Change came later in Germany, where industrialization was a feature of the late 19th century. In England, two-thirds of the population were in large cities by the end of the century. The major industrial cities grew even more rapidly—Birmingham sevenfold between 1800 and 1900 and Hamburg in Germany fivefold between 1850 and 1913.

The response was initially left almost entirely to the market. Housing was overcrowded, with little access to clean water or to sanitation. In London in the 1880s the ratio was forty inhabitants to one privy. Flushing water closets were rare and people might

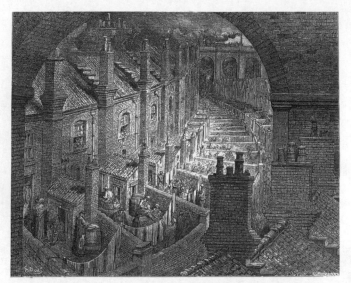

5. This engraving by Gustave Doré shows London with its cramped living conditions and unregulated development. The railway viaduct is built close to workers' housing. Such conditions helped fuel the environmentalism of 19th-century public health.

defecate into pots at home, the contents of which were thrown into watercourses, street drains, or outdoor dung heaps or cesspools. Privies of whatever type would be shared between households, making it difficult to maintain cleanliness. They would have been risky sites for diseases of faecal oral transmission such as typhus and cholera. 'Nuisances'—rubbish and waste—were collected on the streets, and access to clean drinking water was poor. Most housing would not have had piped water. Even as late as 1904, there was one tap per fourteen houses on average in parts of Manchester. Water would be supplied by private contractors from a standpipe and the cost limited consumption. Municipal waterworks, if these existed, could draw water from lakes and sources polluted by sewage.

Epidemics and theories of disease

The 18th century had also had its slum conditions, overcrowding, and fever. But these had not been considered appropriate areas for central government action. This was left to local initiative, to local vestries and parishes in England or to local commissioners who took responsibility for certain local matters such as street cleaning, in return for levying a local rate. This patchwork response was far from the 'medical police' in the continental European countries and it could not cope with the different scale of urban hygiene problems in the 19th century.

The 19th-century public health movement, the motor of a very different state response to public health problems, was traditionally viewed as the response to the series of cholera pandemics of this period. These were indeed a major stimulus, but such a simple disease-focused explanation is not the full one. What also came into play were fears about the potential infection of middle class society from the degraded environment of the urban poor; the growing discussion of the interconnection between poverty, health, and economic development; the role of scientific and in particular statistical investigation; debates about the role of the state; and theories of disease which presupposed particular courses of action. All of this was typical of the 19th-century public health movement, but we can see there issues which have continued to characterize public health responses after the 19th century as well.

Cholera was the initial motor of reform. The first pandemic to reach Europe from India came in 1830, arriving in Sunderland, a port in the north of England, in 1831. It then travelled widely in all directions, reaching London in 1832. Its rapidity of spread and high mortality brought fear to a head. In England and other European countries, cholera brought political unrest in its train. Riots occurred in Russia, France, and England, with the cholera riots of 1831 being directed against doctors, in the belief that the medical profession was encouraging the spread of the disease in order to obtain bodies for dissection. This was also the most violent period of civil disorder during the agitation for political reform which resulted in the 1832 Reform Act. Cholera was spread by social dislocation and subsequently exacerbated it.

Debate about the appropriate response was underpinned by the two main explanations of the spread of epidemic disease: miasmatic and contagious. Miasmatists argued that communal diseases were spread through the air, the result of atmospheric conditions or particles in the air. They paid particular attention to rotting organic matter such as refuse or faeces, anything which smelled badly. Contagionists, on the other hand, argued that diseases were spread from one individual to another. This justified the desire to avoid people with the disease or to quarantine them, and also displayed fears about the origin of disease in working class or other marginalized groups. A middle position, contingent contagionism, argued that diseases might be either miasmatic or contagious, dependent on circumstances. A disease could spread initially through corrupt air but individuals could then become the focus, leading to contagion.

Cholera brought such issues to a head. The initial response across Europe was mostly that of quarantine—along with inspection of people and goods arriving from the infected areas. But after the first epidemic was over it was widely agreed that quarantine had been ineffective. British policy thereafter relied on port inspection and isolation of suspicious cases, covering both theories. Britain opposed quarantine as a method of epidemic control, not least for commercial considerations, although mercantile interests did not always oppose it. Cholera was characterized by broader social and ideological responses as well. It killed the economically vulnerable, reflecting social inequality but also the political culture of the time.

The impact of cholera was variable, not least on either side of the Atlantic. In the United States it gave expression to dominant cultures of religious piety and individualistic voluntarism while in Britain and in most of Europe it heightened social tensions. In the US it did not contribute to any lasting change in public health administration, while in both Britain and France it was an engine of public health reform. Epidemic disease often fulfils this function, depending on the society in which it occurs: we can see this policy and social effect much later with the impact of the HIV/AIDS epidemic.

Public health change

In Britain, the unrest which accompanied cholera also led to a discussion of poverty and its relationship to economic development. This inevitably led to consideration of the relationship between poverty and disease. In the wake of the cholera epidemic, the British government set up a royal commission on the Poor Laws, the long-established local mechanism for dealing with poverty, to examine how the Old Poor Law operated and to make proposals for reform. Established in Elizabethan times, the Poor Law could no longer cope with an urbanized and industrial society. Discussion of reform was informed by the ideas of Thomas Malthus about population growth. Malthus had argued in the late 18th century (1798) that keeping the poor alive could simply amplify poverty later on. Measures to keep poor children alive did no good in the long run. Such arguments have reverberated down the centuries and we hear echoes of them today in discussion of the 'carrying capacity' of poor nations in LICs.

Poor Law reform highlighted the connection between poverty and disease and brought a key figure into public health improvement: Edwin Chadwick. Chadwick, as secretary to the Poor Law Commission, was a dominant figure who straddled the connection between poverty and disease. He was a Benthamite, a follower of the philosopher Jeremy Bentham (1748–1832), whose ideas about the 'greatest happiness of the greatest number' brought Enlightenment beliefs about reason and the perfectibility of man into the realm of the 19th-century reformers. Sanitarianism was the creed which sprang from this doctrine.

The reform of the Poor Law also led to sanitary reform. The new Poor Law of 1834, which was the basis of relief until 1929, operated the principle of less eligibility, that relief should be at a lower rate than that obtainable through paid work. It was hated for its harshness and it led Chadwick down the path of public health reform. In his famous 1842 *Report on the Sanitary Condition of the Labouring Population of Great Britain*, he compiled an extensive survey of the health and living conditions of the poor, through questionnaires and requests submitted to about 2,000 people. His case for reform was compelling but was not based on humanitarianism. He emphasized the benefit to the economy through saving those capable of productive labour; and also the moral benefit of fostering moral and civic decency. This combination of economic and moral determinism has long been a feature of public health—one can trace this combination in public health responses down to the present, where the good health of a population is seen as a component of economic development.

Chadwick's reliance on 'evidence' and the numerical basis of surveys and statistics was typical of the reform movements of the time. Civil registration was introduced in England in 1837, and it became common to quantify the differences in mortality rates and average expectation of years at birth between overcrowded urban areas and rural ones, and between rich and poor. Local sanitary organizations and national campaigning bodies, such as the Health of Towns Association, used statistics as their rationale. This was an international trend. In Paris, the French statistician Louis-René Villermé had adopted the *method numérique* in exploring associations between health and environmental conditions in different *arrondissements* of Paris.

To solve the problem of filth diseases, Chadwick's miasmatic views led him to propose an arteriovenous system of sewage disposal. Essentially, his solution was drains. In 1848, when cholera returned, a General Board of Health was set up with Chadwick as one of its three members. The legislation allowed communities to appoint a Medical Officer of Health (MoH) if 10 per cent of ratepayers petitioned for it. An MoH was compulsory only if the death rate was greater than 23 per 1,000 in the area. But the board was short-lived and was abolished in 1854. Chadwick's dictatorial behaviour caused opposition. There was also widespread resistance to the intervention of the state in such matters. *The Times* famously said that it would rather take its chance with cholera than be bullied into health. Such arguments are echoed in the more recent 'nanny state' discussions about public health.

The use of compulsion also caused opposition in two other areas of public health in the 19th century: vaccination for infectious disease and sexual health. Vaccination is still a key public health tactic, but it has been fraught with concerns about acceptability which its history helps us to understand. It replaced inoculation, which had involved introducing material from the pustules of someone who had the disease into the body of someone who had not. A single episode of disease was recognized to confer lifelong immunity. The procedure, using a scratch in the skin, was introduced to England by Lady Mary Wortley Montagu, wife of the British ambassador in Turkey, after she had seen it in use there.

Edward Jenner, a GP in Gloucestershire, knew that in his area a single episode of cowpox sometimes produced a mild illness in the milkmaids, but they thereafter seemed immune from the more serious smallpox. In 1796, he performed a crucial experiment, building on what others had done locally. He took some matter from a cowpox lesion on the hand of a milkmaid, Sarah Nelmes, and injected it into the arm of a young boy, James Phipps, who had not had natural smallpox. The boy developed some soreness but remained well, and afterwards proved to be immune to smallpox. Jenner published a treatise about the new procedure, called 'vaccination'—after the cow—and the strategy was rapidly taken up by government.

Free vaccination for smallpox was made available through the Poor Law medical services as early as 1840, a very early example of a state-provided service. From the 1850s, vaccination of young children was compulsory and penalties became more severe in a subsequent Vaccination Act of 1867. The Acts were the target of a substantial anti-vaccination movement in Victorian England, which had support across the classes and which achieved a conscientious objection clause in 1907. There were concerns about medical despotism, safety, and the inequitable application of the Acts between rich and poor. The guiding principle was resistance to the growth of government intervention in the civil liberty of the individual.

Compulsory inspection and isolation of prostitutes led to another battle over the enforcement of health. A series of Contagious Diseases Acts were passed in 1864, 1866, and 1869. They were primarily aimed at the eradication of venereal diseases in the army and instituted strict regulation, medical examination, and policing of prostitutes in military areas. However, there were no controls on the men with whom the prostitutes consorted. A campaign against the Acts was led by Josephine Butler and her organization, the Ladies National Association. It stressed not just opposition to compulsion but the 'double standard' of morality which regulated women but not men. This focus on women as a 'public health problem' with a focus on control and on sexuality is something we will see recurring often in public health up to the present day — take for example the recent concerns about women's 'binge drinking' which have ignored the much greater amount of men's drinking.

The Acts were eventually repealed in 1886, not so much out of opposition to compulsion in health policy, but more as part of parliamentary politics of the time. The Acts can be seen in different ways. They demonstrated a new and closer relationship between medicine, public health, and the state. It was also the case that repressive regulation could have health benefits. Cases of neonatal ophthalmia, a side-effect of syphilis, fell during the operation of the Acts. In fact, the second half of the 19th century saw the growth of a public health bureaucracy and greater powers for public health in line with changing views about the role of the state in the regulation and control of many areas. The infectious disease laws created at the end of the 19th century—the notification laws—gave powers to remove sufferers of infectious disease from communities and place them in isolation or fever hospitals. In 1899, an Act made notification compulsory throughout England and Wales.

The universal appointment of a local medical official, the MoH, came after the Public Health Act of 1872. John Simon, Medical Officer initially to the Privy Council Office and then, until 1876, to its successor, the Local Government Board, was a key influence on developments this time around. Advances took place at the local level and were codified in the Public Health Act of 1875. A new cadre of state bureaucrats developed. The MoH was a doctor whose primary function was the provision of health in the community and who relinquished the treatment of illness in individuals. MoHs were responsible for the removal of nuisances, and the implementation of the regulation of lodging houses, building standards, and the condition of bakeries, slaughter houses, and dairies. From the late 1880s they enforced notification and isolation, and by the turn of the century they were supervising local social services such as health visiting.

So far the focus has been on England as the first country to experience industrialization, urbanization, and the public health issues which resulted. But responses in other countries were different and dependent on national variables and country-specific factors. Some countries also produced reports on the model of

Chadwick's in 1842. In the United States, there was John Griscom's *The Sanitary Condition of the Labouring Population in New York* (1845) and Lemuel Shattuck's *Report of the Sanitary Commission of Massachusetts* (1850). But the United States was suspicious of central Federal institutions and so public health action mostly took place at the level of the city or the state. It was only in 1902 that a Federal Public Health and Marine Hospital Service (renamed the US Public Health Service in 1915) was formed, initially as an advisory body to manage immigration. In France, despite its early focus on investigation and statistics, most action also took place at the local level.

Germany was not united until the 1870s, but codified public health law early on, in line with the 'medical police' of the 18th-century states. A central Imperial Hygiene Department was set up in 1873 to collect statistics, control infectious disease, vaccinate for smallpox, and regulate the medical profession. Earlier, in Prussia, the leading German state, during the Europe-wide revolutions of 1848–9, public health reform had been associated with the expression of health as a democratic right, and health reform had been connected with the removal of poverty. Reacting against state policing systems, revolutionary doctors argued that diseases were caused by political repression and economic and educational deprivation.

Rudolf Virchow, a doctor who had spent time on the barricades in Berlin during the revolution, was sent by the authorities to what they hoped was a quiet backwater in Upper Silesia to investigate an epidemic of typhus. His report, *Communications about the Typhus Epidemic in Upper Silesia*, blamed the outbreak on social deprivation, poverty, illiteracy, and political inequality. Democracy and social justice were the best way to control such epidemics in future. He wrote that 'Medicine is a social science, and politics is nothing more than medicine on a large scale.' He subsequently became a distinguished pathologist, but is best known for this stirring defence of the political role of public health.

Virchow's connection between better public health and radical social and political change has informed recent historical interpretations of public health. It represents a dilemma which always confronts public health. Historians have argued that interpretations of public health reform in the 19th century, which see it as 'progress' pure and simple, are deficient. The progressive argument about public health reform sees the adverse effects of economic development gradually set right by a combination of public health interventions, science and evidence, campaigning, and social concern. Change was driven by need.

This is a framework of assumptions which is still used in the public health field today. But it ignores wider and often less altruistic motives. Chadwick made a connection between the good health of the labour force and national industrial development. This 'human capital' argument was taken further by the French philosopher-historian Michel Foucault in his more recent interpretation of public health. To him, public health interventions were an aspect of 'biopolitics', society's control over the body as a force of labour power. Foucault argued that public health primarily benefited the privileged sections of society, protecting them from the threat of epidemic disease and ensuring that the workforce stayed healthy.

Another critique came from the American historian Christopher Hamlin, who has argued that public health in the 19th century took the easy path of the 'technical fix'. He argues:

> the early Victorians invented one public health among many. Their sanitary movement was not a systematic campaign to eliminate excess mortality. Its concern was with some aspects of the health of some people: working class men of working age. Women, infants, children and the aged were largely ignored.... Yet there was another position, a position which viewed as pathological the totality of social and economic conditions in which the Industrial Revolution had left many poor people.... There was here the raw material for

making health as prominent a criterion for the assessment of public policy as, say, economics has become. This did not happen. Chadwick and company rejected work, wages and food to focus on water and filth, arguably the greatest 'technical fix' in history.

Hamlin draws attention to a recurrent issue in public health: that many interventions—for example vaccination—are technical fixes which do little to address more fundamental issues of inequality which have underpinned the development of ill health in the population. They do not alter those fundamentals. Often public health interventions are the 'art of the possible', dependent on time and circumstance.

Germ theory and its diffusion

Chadwick's sanitarianism was underpinned by his belief in miasmatic theories of disease. But in the second half of the 19th century theories of disease began to change, and germ theory became the dominant mode of explanation. Even before this, there had been challenges to miasma which are now recognized as significant, although they were not accepted at the time.

In Bristol, William Budd, Bristol's MoH from 1849, worked on typhoid (salmonella poisoning) and had deduced that polluted water was the cause. John Snow, an ambitious London doctor, anaesthetist, and epidemiologist, is better known for his discoveries about the transmission of disease. He had studied cholera since he was an apprentice in the 1830s and suspected water contaminated by faeces. In 1854 he carried out two classic community experiments which are still used to teach public health students today. The episode of the Broad Street pump is the most famous.

Snow systematically investigated house to house cases of cholera in Soho, London, which had taken water from the pump, and also those further distant (including West Hampstead in north-west

London, where a local widow liked the taste of the Broad Street water and had it carried to her), and incriminated the pump as the source of infection. His dramatic removal of the pump handle was symbolic since the epidemic was already on the wane. His second investigation was a more substantial one, comparing the sickness among people in the same areas who bought their water from different Thames water companies. One supplied filtered water, taken from the Thames upstream. The other supplied it unfiltered and taken lower down in London, complete with sewage. He showed that the people using the unfiltered water had thirteen times the chance of falling ill with cholera than people using the cleaner supplies.

Snow did not succeed in overturning the dominant miasmatic theory, despite the strength of his evidence. That change occurred with the bacteriological revolution of the late 19th century, and was associated with figures such as Robert Koch and Louis Pasteur. The laboratory became an important component of public health, with investigation of the role of microorganisms in disease using microscopy and new techniques of cultivation. Pasteur successfully trialled his rabies vaccine in 1885. Other researchers identified the causal role of different organisms, with Robert Koch's work on anthrax (1876), tuberculosis (1882), and cholera (1883), and Charles Louis Alphonse Laveran's on malaria (1880). The organisms responsible for typhus, diphtheria, tetanus, plague, and dysentery were all discovered. But before the turn of the century knowledge of specific organisms rarely resulted in therapies. It was not until the mid-1890s that two developments of practical value occurred—the use of a diphtheria serum antitoxin and a typhoid vaccine.

Historians have pointed out that this raft of discoveries did not immediately overturn the dominant set of theories held by those in the public health field. There was no instant switch to a new way of thinking. Perhaps the most famous example of this was the opposition of the first German professor of public hygiene, Max von Pettenkofer, to germ theory. His opposition to bacteriology led to a famous showdown with the discoverer of the cholera bacillus, Robert Koch, during the Hamburg cholera epidemic of 1892, when Pettenkofer drank a weakened solution of the bacillus in order to refute Koch's theories. This heroic stance did not dissuade the Hamburg authorities, who followed Koch's instructions to introduce sand filtration of the water supply in order to halt cholera infection in the town.

The new public health at the turn of the century

Despite the initial uneven diffusion of bacteriology, its impact on public health was significant. It underpinned a new style of public health which moved its focus from general improvement of the environment as a whole to the role of the individual, and especially the individual mother, in the home. The success of bacteriology instilled a single-factor explanation for disease, where emphasis was placed on the invading organism, and this brought an expectation of single-factor solutions—magic bullets such as the drug Salvarsan, discovered in 1907 for the treatment of syphilis. The new environmental explanation was the environment of the home rather than the urban environment in general.

This change was underpinned by wider social and economic factors. Towards the end of the 19th century, the balance of economic power was shifting away from Britain and towards Germany and the United States. Fears of economic decline at home and loss of empire abroad were sharpened during the Boer War by revelations about the state of the nation's manpower. The examination of Boer War recruits produced a devastating picture of physical inadequacy. There had been fears since the 1870s about the declining birth rate. The Boer War panic highlighted the 'differential birth rate', the apparently higher rates of conception among what was called the 'residuum', the lower and 'inefficient' (in the language of the time) sections of society. Historians who have examined the data conclude that there was in fact no clear difference in birth rates, but rather significant regional differences which affected all classes. But the national debate was premised on the belief in class differences and expressed the social fears of the time.

Concern also shifted away from infectious diseases in general to what were termed the scourges or 'racial poisons'—tuberculosis, alcoholism, and venereal disease. Mental deficiency too was considered to be a problem because of the threat of national deterioration through transmission and inheritance of these disorders of 'degeneration'. The environmentalist discussions of the mid-century gave way to a strong emphasis on heredity and degeneration of the 'race' coupled with inevitable biological decline. Such theories were common across Europe and in North America, particularly the United States. Herbert Spencer, the British social theorist, advanced theories of 'social Darwinism' which claimed that attempts to ameliorate conditions of social disadvantage had interfered in the natural self-regulation of society and had allowed artificial selection to flourish. Biological degeneration had been facilitated. Theorists such as Cesare Lombroso in Italy based their research on the physiological characteristics of the 'criminal type'.

Eugenics was the creed which resulted, and which was a widely accepted way of thinking about health and society in the early 20th century. Eugenics was a doctrine which united thinkers across a broad spectrum. 'Negative eugenics' focused on tactics such as birth control, sterilization, or segregation of 'the unfit'. Its legacy was ultimately in the racial policies of Nazi Germany. But it was a theory which had a wide appeal in a number of nations, the United States and Sweden for example, in the early decades of the 20th century. The other dimension of eugenics—'positive eugenics'—advanced ideas such as welfare reforms and public health interventions which had the support of social reformers. The institution of legislation for school meals, health insurance, and old age pensions together with compulsory school medical inspection, introduced in 1907 in the UK, owed less to these ideas than to health campaigning and the role of labour.

Anxieties over population quantity and quality stimulated interest in maternal and child welfare. In Britain, as mortality rates for the population as a whole began to decline, those for infant mortality remained high and just before 1900 began to increase. Maternal mortality also remained high into the 1930s. The infant mortality rate was 146 per 1,000 in 1876 and rose to 156 per 1,000 in 1897, an increase of nearly 6.8 per cent. Welfare programmes for mothers and children were strongly advocated by voluntary organizations, for example the Women's Cooperative Guild, which set up some of the first voluntary welfare centres, putting pressure on public health. This led to a greater focus on preventive medicine in the public health profession.

Public health was dependent on changing habits of domestic hygiene, and reinforcing public education. The agenda advocated by the public health service came to include welfare programmes for pregnant and postnatal mothers, infants, and schoolchildren. Different remedies were offered by different factions. George Newman, Medical Officer at the Board of Education, thought the problem was ignorant and feckless mothering, while Arthur Newsholme, CMO of the Local Government Board, saw the solution as the public health management of all community life. Home visiting, inspection, and education of the mother and baby was provided along with milk depots, which gave clean milk and education of the mother in infant feeding. The attitude of mothers to health visiting could be ambivalent. Some historians have argued that health visiting was initially viewed as a police force rather than a resource by poor mothers, who resisted the visitors' advice and dreaded their inspections. But gradually an accommodation was reached.

By the early years of the 20th century, a number of factors had brought a new style of public health which was very different from the environmentalist and sanitarian model of mid-century: the influence of new styles of science (bacteriology and germ theory); new scientific ideologies like eugenics and the focus on inheritance and degeneration; and new economic and social pressures, such as the changes in population and the decline of empire.

Chapter 5
The rise of lifestyle: 1900–1980s

Public health underwent further redefinition during the 20th century. The focus on mothers and babies heightened during World War I, and after the war a 'public health empire' developed in the UK—a range of services run by public health doctors. Historical debates about whether or not this was a wrong turn are relevant to current debates in the public health field. In the interwar years, public health seemed to be a key to the future of national health services, but after World War II this hope proved to be false. The war brought national health and welfare services in many countries, but these were not run by public health, as expected. Changing patterns of disease, known as the *epidemiologic transition*, as well as the changes in health services, also encouraged public health as a profession to seek new avenues. Diseases of lifestyle and chronic diseases were replacing the old pattern of epidemic infectious disease. In the decades after World War II, public health began to pursue a new role in dealing with these population-wide conditions. It was part of a questioning of the authority of clinical medicine which took place in the 1970s.

World War I and after

In Germany, World War I had a considerable impact on health services. During the war, the state accepted its responsibility to maintain the health of the population. Maternity allowances, schemes to improve midwifery services, and health and welfare centres were opened, and condoms as a barrier to STDs were officially sanctioned. In Britain, there was some change but in a more piecemeal way. The pre-existing concern for the health of mothers and babies rose to new heights during the war, and it was argued that it was more dangerous to be a baby than a soldier. Infant mortality was in fact in decline and continued to fall during the war. The number of clinics and health visitors expanded and the 1918 Maternity and Child Welfare Act enabled but did not oblige local authorities to provide services in this area (Figure 6).

But there was increased mortality from tuberculosis, and STDs also spread under wartime conditions. Legislation during and

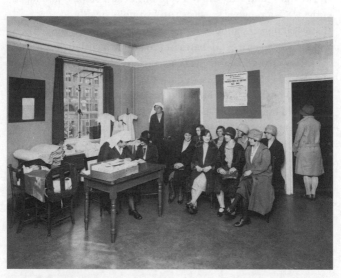

6. In the late 19th century, under the impact of germ theory, public health changed its emphasis to the individual. The role of individual women as mothers was seen as important and many countries passed legislation in the early 20th century to provide mother and baby clinics.

after the war extended provision at the local level both for tuberculosis and for STDs. It was argued during the war that the provision of prophylactics would condone and encourage immorality, and these concerns prevented their distribution in the UK and the US although not in Germany. Such debates paralleled later controversies about whether advice should be given on 'safe sex' during the AIDS era of the 1980s and 1990s. Does providing information and harm-reduction techniques like condoms encourage or prevent certain risky behaviours? The war did result in a network of local authority-run open-access clinics for the treatment of STDs which later formed a basis for the UK response to AIDS.

Alcohol was an area of wartime concern, and in England a Central Control Board was set up in 1915 to direct state policy, which included the provision of state-run public houses in some areas. The work of the board, with its emphasis on direct intervention and also on research and evidence, was a distinct break with pre-war temperance concern about alcohol, which had been separate from the public health movement. The board did not long outlive the war, although its restrictions on pub opening hours lasted until 1987. In the UK alcohol consumption was in decline post-war, and the alcohol issue was no longer central to temperance or part of public health. But elsewhere it was different. Prohibition was instituted in the United States during the 1920s and a 'global prohibition wave' took place which encompassed countries such as Russia, Iceland, Finland, Canada, and Norway. But such prohibition regimes were not long-lived.

The three scourges or 'racial poisons' of the pre-war years—venereal disease, tuberculosis, and alcohol—were of generally decreased importance after the war. The pre-war focus on genetics and heredity was also of lessening importance, although still a strong theme in social and health thinking. Epidemic disease had not departed, and the 1918–19 influenza pandemic brought huge numbers of deaths in its train, perhaps 200,000 in Britain alone.

There were epidemics of typhus and cholera associated with severe famine in Eastern Europe in 1920–2, causing the deaths of many millions. We will look at how public health at the international level expanded to respond to these emergencies in Chapter 6.

Local government services: a location for public health?

In the UK, World War I resulted in the Ministry of Health in 1919 and also in a patchwork of services for special groups and the beginnings of a service empire for public health doctors. The interwar years saw the public health profession at the peak of its professional and service influence. But this also brought dilemmas for public health which have relevance for contemporary debates about where it is best located. It has been argued that public health neglected a 'community watchdog' role in favour of a focus on running services during this period.

Educating the public had been a public health function since the 19th century, and this role expanded markedly in the interwar years. One significant new development was the role of national organizations in the field. In Britain, the Central Council for Health Education was established in 1927, based on the previous British Social Hygiene Council which had focused on venereal diseases. In Leicester in the English Midlands, the local government health committee began to hold health weeks in the 1920s. Posters and handbooks were distributed and there were film screenings. Doctors and nurses gave health talks and there were exhibitions and tea parties. A national health campaign in 1937 included talks, articles in the press, and a public meeting where the audience listened to a radio broadcast by the Prime Minister, Neville Chamberlain.

Public health doctors were also running a widening range of health services. The legislation of the 1870s, in particular the Act of 1875, had given public health control of clean water, sewerage, regulation of streets, highways, and new buildings, health of dwellings, removal of nuisances, inspection of food, suppression of diseases, sanitary burial, regulation of markets, and registration of sickness. Subsequent legislation made different diseases notifiable, required local authorities to supervise the regulation of midwives, established a medical service in schools administered by local government, and gave local authorities the power to provide welfare services for mothers and children and to provide clinics for tuberculosis and venereal disease. The culmination of this trend towards service development under the mantle of public health came with the Local Government Act of 1929, when local authorities were allowed to take over the medical services of the Poor Law. Public health doctors could find themselves in charge of the local hospital and thus also running a range of clinical services.

The profession itself later saw this period as a 'golden age' when it had great power and influence, and the return to local government which took place in England in 2012 was seen as 'coming home'. Historians have been more mixed in their views. Some, writing in the 1980s, saw it as a wrong turn for public health. By taking on such a range of services without a clear idea of what public health was really about, the occupation made itself vulnerable and did not act to improve the health of the poorer sections of the population. Public health doctors were overstretched because of their role in curative health services. There was overlap with the activities of other practitioners, in particular the territory of the general practitioner, a conflict which was portrayed in the battles between the GP, Dr Finlay, and the officious public health doctor, Dr Snoddy, in A. J. Cronin's *Dr Finlay's Casebook*, based on Cronin's own experiences as a GP in a town in Scotland in the late 1920s.

The example of diphtheria immunization supports the 'wrong turn' argument. Effective immunization agents were available by the early 1920s and there were reports of successful trials in Canada and the United States. The British public health profession remained mistrustful of the new approach and concentrated on confining victims in hospital—an old-style quarantine approach. This meant that the death rate in Canada fell in the 1920s and 1930s whereas in Britain there was no decline until the 1940s, after the initiation of a national immunization scheme in 1941.

Few in the public health field took up the issue of the effect of long-term unemployment on nutritional standards and mortality and morbidity rates. G. C. M. McGonigle, the MoH for Stockton on Tees, was one of the small number of public health doctors who were involved. In his book, *Poverty and Public Health* (1936), he reported that the death rate among poor families was twice that for the more affluent. But the lead in raising such questions came largely from outside the public health profession, by political lobbying groups such as the Children's Minimum Council, the Committee against Malnutrition, and the National Unemployed Workers' Movement, all of which called for a higher level of unemployment benefit to enable families to secure minimal nutritional requirements. Richard Titmuss, an insurance clerk, self trained as a social scientist and later Professor at the London School of Economics, conducted a survey of infant mortality and concluded that the decline in infant mortality was not accompanied by a narrowing of the gap between the classes. Obstetricians and gynaecologists also drew attention to high maternal mortality and morbidity rates. A new scientific discipline, nutrition, appeared on the scene. In *Food Health and Income* (1936) the nutritionist John Boyd Orr showed that one-tenth of the population and one-fifth of children were ill-nourished.

The dilemma was the same as it had been for 19th-century public health: should public health as a profession and body of knowledge have played a greater role in advancing social justice at a time of high unemployment? Recent historical research has presented a more nuanced and perhaps less critical picture of the role of public health in these years. It has showed how there was vitality at the local level and how local circumstances could determine decisions about what expenditure there was on public health activity. There were variations in expenditure at the local level which suggest that room existed for local councils and officers to set priorities for spending according to local need within the constraints imposed by national and fiscal factors. Party politics may have determined those decisions at the local level, but it is clear that the role of key individuals pursuing policy objectives in local settings was also important. A strong-minded MoH working within political structures could achieve improved public health outcomes.

There is currently more cause for optimism in assessing interwar public health work. The newer interpretation argues that running health services was not a diversion for public health. Rather, it started to bring together preventive and curative services. The influence of a high-profile local official, the MoH, could be considerable. The annual health report brought together health statistics on the area. The MoH headed a well-staffed department with workers ranging from health visitors to sanitary inspectors. There was a threefold decrease in infectious disease mortality rates, from around 350 per 100,000 population in 1917 to 150 per 100,000 in 1937, to reach 10–20 per 100,000 in 1957.

Social medicine

Such debates draw attention to the continuing dilemmas facing public health in terms of its location, ideology, and core activities. The breadth of topics and initiative embodied in public health make the dilemmas unresolvable. A new vision for public health came on to the agenda of some countries and on to the international scene in the interwar years. Out of the older ideas of 'social hygiene' came novel ways of thinking about the relationship between medicine and social factors, and the integration of prevention and curative approaches. These became known as 'social medicine', a term which is still used in public health circles. The term can be traced as far back as the 1830s in France, and it has had many meanings over time.

Its genesis in the 20th century is associated with Soviet Russia. Social hygiene departments set up in Russian universities after the revolution, and the training of doctors, were based on those principles. Health and disease were seen as expressions of socio-economic inequality. There was also a tradition from the time of the tsars of understanding social influences on disease. Both traditions in Russian society believed that the improvement of material conditions would result in lower disease and death rates. Soviet social medicine placed a high priority on preventive medicine, and preventive health care was linked with the promotion of positive health. There were innovative experiments with birth control clinics, child guidance clinics (incorporating psychoanalysis), and cosmetic services for sufferers from facial cancers and other disfiguring illnesses.

In both Europe and the United States, there were attempts to create a new academic discipline of social medicine. Enthusiastic proponents promoted the approach in both the United States and in Britain. At Yale University in the 1930s, an Institute of Human Relations was founded to bring together medicine and social issues. In Britain, an Institute of Social Medicine was founded at Oxford University in 1942, with the idea that social medicine would be the foundation of medical training after the war. John Ryle, the first professor of social medicine at Oxford, wrote that health was the 'whole economic, nutritional, occupational, educational and psychological opportunity or experience of the individual or community'. The movement was strong in France and Belgium. In Belgium, the Rockefeller Foundation funded a chair of social medicine in 1945 held by the social medicine pioneer René Sand. It was confidently expected that such ideas could form the basis of public health and its role in health services in the post-war world.

Public health after World War II: changed circumstances and new definitions

The changes expected to be driven by public health did not happen, however, and public health underwent a further redefinition after the end of the war. One factor underpinning this redefinition was the changing pattern of disease (Figure 7).

Overall mortality for both males and females from infectious diseases declined precipitately, with a slight increase in deaths among males from the late 1980s (related to HIV/AIDS). The pattern of mortality from cancer and circulatory diseases was more complex, with a general increase in their proportionate importance by comparison with the great killer epidemics of the past. These were diseases which could be linked to behaviours rather than to infections or polluted environments.

Another post-war change was the rise of collective responsibility for health care. Between 1945 and 1964, all sixteen countries in Western Europe greatly extended responsibility for health care. Most of the services were components of compulsory insurance-based schemes for social security developed from Prussian social security reforms instigated under Bismarck. They involved a connection between payments and benefits. In Britain, a different type of system, primarily tax-funded, was put into operation in 1948. Public health and its pre-war 'empire' had originally been intended to be the lynchpin of the new service. But the political realities of bringing the service into existence meant that its focus was rather the voluntary elite hospitals and the specialist system of health care. Public health was sidelined by the determination of hospital consultants. Locally, the GP gradually took over many of the functions of the old MoH. The NHS was a 'sickness' rather than a positive health focused service from the start.

Public health both as an occupation and as a body of knowledge was left struggling to find a new role. The idea that social

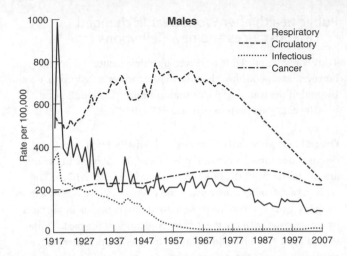

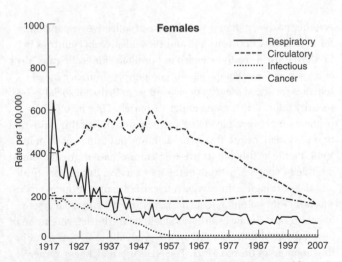

7. After World War II, changes in mortality were apparent, with a decreasing proportion of deaths from infectious disease and a rise in the importance of diseases of 'lifestyle' such as cancer and heart disease. Public health changed its own focus in response to this epidemiological transition.

medicine would be the foundation of health services proved doomed. Only in some countries did its ideas live on post-war. In India, the Bhore Committee looked towards the establishment of a health system that emphasized preventive measures and was based on salaried workers in a public health service which linked villages to district health centres. In South Africa, the Gluckman Commission had a similar rationale and social medicine ideas animated the Karks in their establishment of the Pholela primary health care clinic in the 1940s in KwaZulu-Natal.

What emerged from the ruins of social medicine was a new focus on diseases of behaviour or 'lifestyle', on chronic disease, and on the role of quantitative techniques to investigate these behaviours. The technical tools used were those of chronic disease epidemiology with ideas about 'risk' and 'risk factors' for disease. Thus rather than investigating the direct causation of disease through infection or germs, public health personnel began to focus on the role of long-term risk factors which might not cause disease immediately but might eventually bring ill health in the future. They began to use a new language: that of 'lifestyle'—that is, of individual behaviour or habits—and how this might be modified. This brought, as we will see, a whole new way of operating for public health.

A key text which epitomized the change in public health came from a social medicine pioneer active since the 1930s. In 1957, Jerry Morris, a doctor and epidemiologist with strong social medicine sympathies, published *Uses of Epidemiology*, a text which underpinned the new approach. Morris had worked closely with Richard Titmuss in the 1930s and 1940s when they had published important studies of the relationship between occupation, class, and health. In the 1950s, his work changed its emphasis. An occupational study of rates of heart disease among bus drivers and bus conductors revealed that these were higher among the sedentary drivers than the active conductors. The explanation was lifestyle and exercise. The conductors spent their working lives running up and down the stairs of London's double-decker buses collecting fares. The study originated in the older focus on class and occupational health but its results helped to determine the new focus on lifestyle and behaviour.

Smoking was the issue which epitomized the new approach. In both Britain and the United States, it emerged as a key health issue in the post-war years. The pioneering research was carried out by Richard Doll and Sir Austin Bradford Hill at the London School of Hygiene and Tropical Medicine, as well as by Wynder and Graham in the United States. The rise in deaths from lung cancer led the British Medical Research Council to commission the two scientists to investigate the causes. Their original theory was that it could be to do with the tarring of the roads. A questionnaire delivered to cancer patients in London hospitals revealed that heavy smoking was present in those with lung cancer but not in those with other forms of cancer. The American study found similarly. Doll and Hill then designed a prospective study, following the health of more than 34,000 British doctors, and relating their chances of acquiring lung cancer to their smoking habits. The final report from the study was published in 2005, written by Doll himself and his long-term collaborator Richard Peto. By then the health hazards of smoking were widely accepted.

In more recent times, it has been pointed out that the connection they made was known before the war. The Nazis, with their murderous ideas about racial hygiene, had espoused opposition to tobacco and alcohol based on German research. But these ideas carried little weight because of their origin. The publication of the Royal College of Physicians (RCP) report, *Smoking and Health*, in 1962 was the first to bring the issue to worldwide attention, aided by the new feature of television coverage, and was followed two years later by the US Surgeon General's report on the same subject. The RCP report had originally intended to look at air pollution as well as smoking. But this was left out of the final report because it raised more difficult issues, both in terms of the science and of policy, and possible conflicts with industry. Smoking was an individual habit, which could be more easily dealt with, or so it was thought at the time.

This new way of looking at health issues also encompassed heart disease, food, and diet. In the United States, the Framingham study of heart disease was the best known of the new type of cohort studies, a study with two groups of people with similar characteristics, one of whom receives a treatment or is exposed to a risk factor, while the other is not. The rate of cardiovascular disease had increased in the United States since 1940 by 40 per cent and new theories drew attention to the role of diet in heart disease. The Framingham study began in 1948 and is still ongoing. In 1961, it was the first to use the term 'risk factor'. Research appeared which suggested that diet was a major cause of the rise of coronary heart disease in the Western world. The physiologist and epidemiologist Ancel Keys argued that the Western diet was to blame, with its high levels of saturated fat. Despite scientific debate on this point, the idea gained ground among the health professions of industrialized countries. The American Heart Association was one of the first medical associations to publish guidance for the public on diet in relation to heart disease, with *Food for your Heart* in 1952 and later *Diet and Heart Disease* in 1965 and 1968.

The older public health tactics of inspection, quarantine, and vaccination had little relevance to this changed situation. In the 1960s and 1970s public health developed a new style of operating. There was increased emphasis on the role of the mass media, television in particular, and of health education campaigns that reached out to the whole population. The older tradition of 'health weeks' and talks was replaced by the work of central health education agencies. In Britain, the local authority-funded Central Council for Health Education was replaced by the Health

Education Council in 1968, relaunched in 1973. These agencies used mass media campaigns drawing on advertising agencies and psychological and behavioural insights to reach out and influence the behaviour of populations. The art of 'persuasion' was central, drawing on American-inspired advertising theory (Figure 8).

Epidemiologists such as Geoffrey Rose, at the London School of Hygiene and Tropical Medicine, justified what became known as the 'whole population' approach for public health. The strategies which focused only on high-risk individuals had a limited ability to reduce disease in the whole community. Ultimately, he wrote, 'the only acceptable answer is the mass strategy, whose aim is to shift the whole population's distribution of the risk variable'. The 'whole population' approach underpinned the new style of public health which developed a distinctive way of operating, drawing on the ideas of the emergent profession of health economics, and the disciplines of psychology and sociology. This view did not fit well with the interests of industries such as food or alcohol, which preferred to concentrate on individuals who were 'diseased' or 'high risk'. During the 1970s, opposition between public health interests and industries grew, after an earlier period of cooperation. A public health standard package for policy action was established. This involved demands for increased taxation; mass media health education campaigns; restrictions on advertising of the product; and resolute opposition to cooperation with industry.

Smoking was the issue which first epitomized these developments. In the United States, because of the less centralized nature of the state, the public health community expressed their hostility to industry through legal cases which secured compensation from industrial interests. The new style of public health stimulated criticism about the 'nanny state'. Was it the role of governments to lecture the public about their individual habits? Critics also

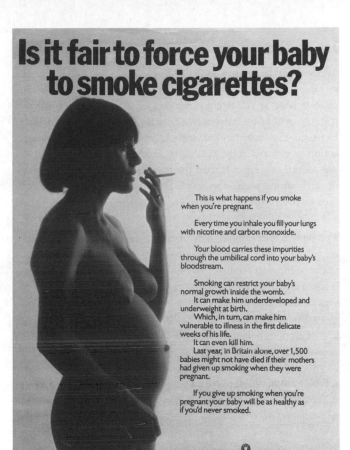

Is it fair to force your baby to smoke cigarettes?

This is what happens if you smoke when you're pregnant.

Every time you inhale you fill your lungs with nicotine and carbon monoxide.

Your blood carries these impurities through the umbilical cord into your baby's bloodstream.

Smoking can restrict your baby's normal growth inside the womb.
It can make him underdeveloped and underweight at birth.
Which, in turn, can make him vulnerable to illness in the first delicate weeks of his life.
It can even kill him.
Last year, in Britain alone, over 1,500 babies might not have died if their mothers had given up smoking when they were pregnant.

If you give up smoking when you're pregnant your baby will be as healthy as if you'd never smoked.

The Health Education Council

8. The new style of public health focused on 'persuasion', using advertising techniques and the mass media. Campaigns developed by the agency Saatchi and Saatchi for the Health Education Council in the UK broke new ground in the 1970s.

cast doubt on the research which proved the connection between lifestyle and ill health. For example ulcers, thought at one stage to arise from poor diet, were later proved to be caused by an infection which could be treated.

The fragmentation of public health

Although public health had found a new role in the post-war world, its range and style of activities was more fragmented. It became characterized by 'single issue' campaigns which used innovative techniques of health advocacy. These techniques derived from the consumer movement in the United States and from the housing action movement in the UK. ASH, established in the UK in 1971, was an early example. It used the mass media in a conscious way through 'stunts' such as buying shares in a tobacco company, and then turning up at the AGM to create a scene.

This new style of campaigning organization did not have the mass membership which temperance had had in the 19th century. It operated through publicity, recognizing it to be crucial in a society increasingly framed around the mass media. The role of advocacy organizations helped to create the conditions for cultural change around smoking and other behavioural issues. They operated as part of a 'policy balancing act', which enabled governments to resist the blandishments of other policy players such as the tobacco industry by drawing attention to opposition to the industry line. Advocacy took different forms in other countries, for example in Australia the AIDS and later Cancer Councils funded both research and advocacy.

The style of operation was far from the service basis of public health before the war. The relationship between public health and health services was problematic in the post-war decades. A new definition of public health within health services was beginning to emerge in the 1960s. This was the concept of 'community medicine' and the 'community physician' who replaced the MoH in the UK. The twin components of the redefined concept were epidemiology and medical administration, and the idea was that the public health doctor would operate as the coordinator or manager of health services. Meanwhile the public health service empire of the interwar years underwent further attenuation. Separate social work departments were set up in local government in the late 1960s, and in 1974 public health doctors moved as community consultants into the NHS. But this move was a poisoned chalice. The arrival of health service general management as a separate non-public health profession in the 1980s undermined the role of coordination intended for public health; and the location in health services took public health doctors away from involvement with their local community.

Meanwhile the GP occupied territory which had once been that of public health, and took on some of the newer public health interventions. Screening was one example: cervical screening, offered from the 1960s, was located in general practice and not in public health. Family planning and prescribing the new contraceptive pill, which became free on prescription in 1974, were also matters for the GP not the public health doctor. Campaigns for women's health were not initiated by public health personnel and the campaign for abortion law reform which resulted in the Abortion Act of 1967 was led by the Abortion Law Reform Association, in existence since the 1930s, not by public health doctors.

Not all countries followed the same patterns—in the United States for example, chronic disease as a concept had greater purchase before World War II and the influence of social medicine was less. But in general the change in focus towards cancer and heart disease and other conditions was common in most developed countries at this time.

Social medicine and evidence-based medicine

Evidence-based medicine was another legacy of social medicine. It was central to post-war moves to make medicine more effective and to apply quantitative techniques to evaluate what it did. The doctor-epidemiologist and social medicine pioneer Archie

Cochrane's lecture and book, *Effectiveness and Efficiency* (1972), helped initiate the movement to research health services and to make them more effective through the application of 'evidence'. Cochrane himself had been closely involved in social medicine in the 1930s. During the Spanish Civil War he had served as a member of a British ambulance unit, and during World War II he was medical officer in a number of prisoner of war camps. These experiences had a profound effect on his future practice of medicine. After the war he joined the Medical Research Council's Pneumoconiosis Unit at Llandough Hospital near Cardiff. Here he began a work on the population of Rhondda Fach—studies which pioneered the use of randomized controlled trials (RCTs). This stimulated an international movement for evidence-based medicine, with advocates in Canada and the United States, and which was also important in the study of health services in the Netherlands. The RCT became seen as the 'gold standard' of such research, leading eventually to the establishment of the Cochrane Centre and collaboration, which developed an international body of evidence.

This was the way in which public health saw its role in relation to health services. Research and evidence became more common as the potential basis for action in other areas of public health. Advocacy groups drew on research, as did government. Sometimes they used evidence which led to differing conclusions, which was the case with research reports on alcohol in the UK at the end of the 1970s. A wider range of research-based disciplines entered the academic public health field—health economics, psychology, and medical sociology. Psychology in particular informed models of behaviour change. But academic public health remained separate from the public health profession. In the UK the profession was almost entirely medical and located in health services. So the fragmentation of public health occurred at many levels: academic public health was separate from service-based public health; medical and non-medical public health did not work together; formal public health occupations such as 'community physicians' and those working in public health occupations such as health advocacy occupied different terrains.

Health inequalities and public health

This fragmentation embodied dilemmas for public health about what its role should be—the same dilemmas it had faced in the mid-19th century. Health inequalities re-emerged in the 1970s as an issue and illustrated some of these difficulties. The concept of 'relative deprivation' was the new way of expressing the role of inequality in industrialized societies.

The Black Report on inequality and health, published in 1980, provided a case study. Commissioned by the Labour government in the 1970s, it was presented to an incoming Conservative government under Margaret Thatcher as Prime Minister. Its recommendations were not acceptable to the new government and it was published in only a limited number of copies on a bank holiday. The resultant media outcry gained the report wide publicity and a subsequent report, *The Health Divide* (1987)—the final report of the Health Education Council before it was subsumed into a new Health Education Authority focused on HIV/AIDS—also attracted attention.

The 'received view' of the rejection of the report was that its conclusions about inequality did not suit the agenda of the Conservative government. But there was also another aspect to the report. Some of the leading researchers on the Black committee were riven by disagreement as to whether its recommendations should focus on services or on initiatives in the community. These disagreements also delayed the submission of the report and hence its impact. They marked a classic dilemma for public health about the 'art of the possible'. In other countries, the inequalities issue was less prominent; in the US discussions were about race rather than class.

Challenges to health services: the McKeown debate on the impact of public health

The 1970s, which had seen the rise of 'whole population' ideas and of lifestyle and behavioural public health, also saw a gathering attack on the efficacy of formal health services. The optimism about high-tech medicine which had marked the immediate post-war years was in decline. This was the outcome of economic factors: the rise in oil prices; uncertainty about how health services could be funded; and criticism of the inappropriate role of high-tech medicine in developing countries. The attack was led by social theorists such as Ivan Illich and Thomas Szasz. It also drew on a critique of the role of public health which has reverberated down the years.

Thomas McKeown, a social medicine academic at the University of Birmingham, used the history of disease and its decline in the 19th and 20th centuries to make his case. He argued that the decline of mortality in the 19th century had not resulted from changing disease virulence or medical technology. Reduced exposure to disease by sanitary intervention played some part, but the decline was mainly due to better nutrition and rising living standards in the second half of the 19th century. The argument about nutrition was one by exclusion—that is, after excluding all other factors, nutrition was the explanation which was left.

In the 1980s, the demographic historian Simon Szreter challenged McKeown's argument. He focused on the role of respiratory tuberculosis. Through re-examination of the statistics, he disputed the contention that tuberculosis was the first disease to decline and that the large group of airborne diseases was as significant as McKeown had claimed in the chronology of the decline of mortality. This meant a reinstatement of the role of the classic hygiene diseases amenable to improvements in sanitation and a reassessment of the role of public health.

This was not simply an abstruse debate about statistics, but one with implications for the decades during which it took place. McKeown had initially represented some of the concerns about formal medicine and public health which preoccupied critics in the 1970s. But his argument was used in the 1980s in developing countries by external funders to justify a central role for economic growth rather than the provision of state infrastructure and intervention, although McKeown himself had not intended this. Szreter's argument was also put forward in the late 1980s when public health was resurgent, and encouraged reconsideration of its potential role in society and the role of the state. This is an ongoing historical debate in which other historians are actively involved in seeking to modify these arguments, and remains of central importance for discussion of the role of public health and the state in societies.

One reason for the resurgence of public health at the end of the 1980s at both national and international levels was the resurgence of infectious disease, epitomized above all by the arrival of HIV/AIDS as an urgent issue on the agendas of both developed and developing countries. In Britain, HIV brought in its train a new role for public health which was underlined in the Acheson Report mentioned in Chapter 1. The subsequent panic about the spread of BSE/nvCJD in the 1980s and 1990s underlined the re-emergence of potential epidemics on the public health agenda and also, in the case of BSE, the growing interconnection between issues of animal and human health. The end of the 20th century and the early years of the 21st saw growing overlap in issues across the world. By the end of the 1970s, public health was undergoing further charge, with new approaches called health promotion and new public health. These were also international movements, and we will look at them in Chapter 6.

Chapter 6
Tropical and international public health

So far the history of public health in this book has mostly concentrated on the rise of public health in what used to be termed 'developed countries', sometimes nowadays termed the 'global North' or high income countries. Now we will look at the establishment of a distinctive tropical public health tied to colonial concerns in the years before World War I; and at the history of public health action at the international level, the precursor of the 'global public health' introduced in Chapter 2.

Public health in the tropics before World War I

Over time, the tropics were separated as areas of study from the European zones in which scientific knowledge was produced. A key linking theme was the role of colonial experience. Whatever the role of different climactic conditions, the experience of being a colony united many of these countries. European exploration in the 15th century and the growth of mercantile empires in the 17th and 18th centuries gave rise to the need to understand exotic societies. The development of cartography, geography, taxonomy, and sciences of classification in the 18th and 19th centuries gave Europeans a way of looking at global biological variety and difference.

Specific concerns arose with the increasing migration of Europeans to new imperial territories. For much of the 19th century, European residence in the tropics was confined to small trading garrisons. Even in India the British East India Company managed British trading and military concerns largely through Indian agency until the Crown assumed control of the government after the Indian Rebellion of 1857. As the remit of the Empire grew, so did concerns about the health of Europeans living among their colonial subjects. Initially in India, for example, there were sanitary reforms similar to those in British cities from the 1830s. But these were confined to military cantonments and to the European quarters of Indian cities.

Vaccination against smallpox was the exception to this European focus. This began in India in 1802, and was performed on Indians relatively early on. As in England, its extension was justified on the grounds of economic efficiency. The extension of vaccination to rural areas of India in the 1820s and 1830s also occurred at a time of reforms in India's administration and was promoted by Benthamite administrators such as Lord Elphinstone, Governor General of Bombay. But its success was relatively limited. There was resistance from the Indian population, which had its own system of inoculation and which often regarded arm to arm vaccination as ritually polluting: people from whom the vaccine was transferred were usually 'untouchables' or other low-caste Indians. The vaccination programme did not reach substantial numbers of Indians until the late 19th century. Again, the importance of understanding local beliefs and circumstances emerges in this instance, as in the case of anti-vaccinationism in the UK.

Increasingly the situation and health of the indigenous population was seen, as in India, as part of the public health problem rather than as a potential example to help facilitate acclimatization to the tropics. The British became more separate from the Indians, whose racial differences were emphasized. There are parallels with the fear of the working class in the public health movement in the UK. Indian dwellings were seen as potential threats to the health of Europeans and there was increasing pessimism about the potential for Europeans to adapt to the tropics. When the government did begin to intervene more directly in public health administration after the Indian Rebellion, it was largely to protect the health of British troops—always a key driver of public health reform. In garrisons, better hygiene and a reduction in overcrowding in the mid-19th century were the key to improved military mortality in tropical conditions.

Tropical medicine

Europeans had begun to acquire a knowledge of the diseases of warm climates, based on a mixture of European and indigenous medical knowledge, but this knowledge was not institutionalized. From the 1880s and the rise of the political culture of imperialism, demonstrated by the 'scramble for Africa', this began to change. The rapid developments in microbiology in Europe—the discovery of 'germ theory' which we examined in Chapter 4—shed light on models of disease transmission in the tropics. Outbreaks of bubonic plague in India and Brazil, sleeping sickness in Central Africa, and Chagas' disease in northern Brazil, presented problems to those concerned with labour, public health, and international trade.

Research attention shifted to the opportunities offered by tropical disease. The patronage of business and government interests associated with the imperialism of the late 19th century gave rise to institutions across the world which were devoted to the new specialism. The Liverpool and London Schools of Tropical Medicine (Hygiene was added to the name of the London School in the 1920s) opened in 1899, while institutes of tropical medicine were founded in Hamburg and Paris in 1901 and Brussels in 1906. Chairs in tropical diseases and medicine were endowed in Harvard and New Orleans in the United States, reflecting both the climactic diversity of the US and its expanded imperial role after the Spanish–American War of 1898.

Malaria was a particular source of morbidity and mortality in the tropics. The early work of the Liverpool School focused on anti-malarial programmes, which attempted to control the disease by the elimination of its vector the *Anopheles* mosquito, discovered by Ronald Ross, the first director of the Liverpool School. Other microorganisms causing cholera, brucellosis, sleeping sickness, bubonic plague, and leishmaniasis were all discovered in the years between 1880 and 1918. But Ross's mentor, Patrick Manson, the driving force behind the emergence of tropical medicine as a distinct speciality, also recognized that it was a label of convenience representing the political as well as the medical needs arising from European imperial activities. Some historians have dismissed these activities as completely self-serving, aimed solely at protecting the health of the European settlers. Others have argued for subtler interpretations, where enlightened self-interest dictated that the health of all had to be considered.

Interventions were, however, geared to the needs of the colonial state. Public health was part of colonial governance. Africans, according to Megan Vaughan, were 'an undifferentiated mass, part of a dangerous environment which needed to be controlled and contained'. The 'great campaigns' against sleeping sickness showed this clearly. From the end of the 19th century up to World War I, latex from wild rubber was a key commodity in European and North American industry. In equatorial Africa, the brutal labour conditions in rubber collection weakened populations and exposed them to the uncleared forest habitats of the tsetse fly. Epidemic sleeping sickness flourished across Central and West Africa and across the Great Lakes region of East Africa, engaging the scientific attention of researchers from France, Belgium, and Portugal.

Two control approaches emerged which characterized tropical medicine in this period, and which continued to inform approaches to the control of epidemic disease. Research on vector control and insect habitat was initiated by the British as a means of interrupting disease transmission by eliminating the insect from the disease cycle. In British East Africa and northern Nigeria, the vector control approach was worked out to its fullest extent. Later, after 1910, French missions to equatorial Africa took a different tack, using systematic case detection, population screening, and the administration of arsenicals, eliminating the parasite from the host. This was the contrast between ecological/entomological and population screening approaches to disease control. In the Belgian Congo, where the former approach was used, the military-style organization of the campaigns was impressive.

Missionary medicine and public health

Missionary medicine had a different public health ethos in sharp contrast to the militaristic and coercive campaigns of early tropical medicine. John Manton writes that 'the impact of Christian missionary medical work on public health was central to overall health care provision'. In most areas of colonial Africa before 1918 up to the 1930s, medical missions were the means by which indigenous peoples experienced Western health care. These were the first to introduce rural health care, and they began to train Africans as midwives and rural health workers. Their main research role was in the area of leprosy control, and their critical contribution was a focus on the conditions of poverty and their local and rural work. The missionary concern for spiritual as well as practical health issues 'represented a wide range of apparently altruistic concerns with welfare and public health in the tropical latitudes'.

Ideas of degeneration and heredity impacted in the tropics as they did in developed countries. But the idea of 'race' and its intersection with public health was of particular significance in the tropics. Ideas of the dying race, or of racial immunity among some populations, were common. Nowhere was this focus on race more obvious than in considerations of sexuality and disease. The conceptual and diagnostic confusion surrounding leprosy, yaws, and syphilis was common. The problem was seen to lie in uncontrolled African sexuality and in particular female sexuality, a discourse also familiar in discussion of the underclass in Victorian Britain. In Africa, it was transformed by the particular circumstance of colonial rule; the sexuality of African peoples became a focus of European concern and representative of the problems of maintaining social order in a rapidly changing society. The needs of colonial governance also on occasion brought different models of control in the colonies to those which operated in the mother country. Hong Kong had wide-ranging Contagious Disease Acts together with state brothels and legalized prostitution which lasted until 1934. In countries such as Uganda, the STD services formed the basis of later national health services.

International health action up to World War II

As we saw in Chapter 3, international efforts to control epidemic disease such as plague and cholera spreading worldwide in earlier centuries had relied on quarantine and closing borders. But in the 19th century ideas and tactics changed, and international public health cooperation based on science was established through embryonic international health organizations. In the century between the Congress of Vienna in 1815 and the outbreak of World War I in 1914, wide-ranging international cooperation emerged in many areas—law, economics, labour, religious and intellectual movements, social and welfare organizations, and humanitarian causes.

International health cooperation had its beginnings in a series of international sanitation conferences which took place between 1851 and 1903. The conferences were stimulated by the spread of epidemic diseases, especially cholera and yellow fever.

The pandemics of 1830 and 1847 had been facilitated by the increased movement of goods and people between East and West and by developments in international commerce, steamships, railways, and later the construction of the Suez Canal. The traditional modes of epidemic control proved difficult to maintain in this era of international commerce. The conventions and regulations emerging from these conferences were never successfully ratified by governments, until the eleventh conference in Paris in 1903 produced the first effective treaty. This formed the basis of a convention which covered quarantine on land and sea up until World War II.

The Paris meeting also took forward the idea of an international coordinating mechanism; the Office International D'Hygiene Publique (OIHP) was established at a meeting in Rome in 1907. It was based in Paris but maintained close cooperation with local 'sanitary councils'; its main function was the collation and dissemination of epidemiological intelligence through a monthly bulletin. Governments were obliged to inform the Office of steps they were taking to implement the sanitary conventions and the office could suggest modifications. It was under the control of a committee composed of one delegate from each participating state, with voting power related to the amount subscribed. It prefigured the organizational structure of later international health bodies, such as the WHO.

The establishment of the OIHP marked a point of transition from international health meetings and conventions to more permanent international health organizations. In 1903 the Pan American Sanitary Bureau was the first of these. Other international issue-based organizations had also come into existence in the 19th century, for example the International Committee of the Red Cross in 1864. Congresses on alcohol led to the formation of an International Temperance Bureau in 1906 which mingled moral concern and science. The same was the case with the International Central Bureau for the Campaign against

Tuberculosis (1902), which emerged from a series of international conferences on tuberculosis which began in the 1860s. The country-based concern about these public health problems and diseases transferred into the international arena.

During the early decades of the 20th century, organizations such as the Rockefeller Foundation, the League of Nations Health Organization (LNHO), and the International Labour Organization (ILO) formed part of an emerging vision of international public health. The years before World War I witnessed the establishment of a new form of international philanthropy, characterized by the Rockefeller Foundation and other mainly US-based institutions—the Millbank Memorial Fund, Commonwealth Fund, and Sage Foundation.

Rockefeller had pioneered a hookworm programme in the southern US before the outbreak of war, and its success had prompted the foundation's strategists to promote hookworm research and treatment across Latin America, providing governments with public health funding and the promise of 'capacity building' in training and developing indigenous expertise. Similar work was carried out in the Philippines. This promise rarely came to pass, and Rockefeller programmes were accused of diluting state sovereignty over health services and projecting US power based on technocratic solutions. Its International Health Board advanced scientific solutions, as for example in Mexico in the hookworm campaign in the 1920s, with the aims also of improving economic productivity and promoting good relations between the US and Mexico. It had an economic and strategic rationale as well as a public health one. The issues raised by its activities are still very relevant to the discussion of the role of international health foundations in the present.

Rockefeller pursued a much more interventionist programme than the US government itself was willing to countenance at this time, just after World War I. It established an International

Health Commission in 1913 and supported clinics, training schemes, and schools of public health and laboratory services throughout the world. It has been common for historians to represent its activities as a stalking horse for American imperialism. More recently, however, their assessment of its role has been more mixed. Undoubtedly American political interests were furthered by its involvement in the League of Nations and in programmes in the Far East and Latin America. But research on Australia and the Pacific Islands has shown that there was no simple imposition of an American model on local populations but a more complex process of bargaining and compromise.

The foundations were relatively free and without public and political constraints. For example, in the aftermath of WWI Rockefeller helped to support a system of socialized primary health care in Serbia. Also in the interwar years, through Rockefeller influence, instruments developed in the US to measure community health performance were transferred to Europe and put to use there. Through its focus on training and institution-building it was crucial in the creation of a network of public health experts based on science, technology transfer, and the exchange of personnel, a model which has endured in international and global public health.

At the end of World War I, the Treaty of Versailles brought a new international organization into being: the League of Nations. The League of Nations had technical agencies with responsibility for health: the ILO and the LNHO. Initially the ILO had a grand vision of its role in health, based on the treaty, which assigned it the role of protecting 'the worker against sickness, disease and injury arising from his [*sic*] employment'. But this broad vision gave way to a narrower approach based on the role of scientific expertise and laboratory proof. So the ILO became a technical organization anchored in the production of scientific evidence about the health effects of particular hazards. No attempt was made to correlate economic trends with the mortality and morbidity data in its labour statistics.

The LNHO, responsible for public health and social medicine, showed a similar narrowing of focus, signalled by its separation from the Social Section of the League of Nations in 1920. The LNHO's main concern in the 1920s was standard-setting, in order to apply scientific principles in a universal way through biological standards and mortality and morbidity statistics. By 1937, over 70 per cent of the world's population was covered by LNHO statistics. This did provide leverage for broader discussion of health and the economy during the depression of the 1930s. Cooperative programmes were developed with the ILO which looked at how diet, housing, and economic conditions shaped health. Areas such as nutrition were particularly lively, as British scientists criticized their government's inaction by invoking nutritional standards endorsed by the LNHO/ILO and forced it to raise the minimum standards used in calculating unemployment and maternity benefits.

The existence of the organization helped in the transfer of ideas about health and social welfare from the US to Europe during the interwar years. 'Unpopular issues' such as STDs were kept at arm's length and were largely taken up by voluntary organizations. The ILO focused mostly on the economically productive sections of the population—not older people, the disabled, or mentally ill—and the LNHO avoided the controversial area of birth control. In one area, that of illicit drugs, a separate international system for control of trade, although in the interests of health, was set up in the interwar period, also initially as part of the Treaty of Versailles. A series of international conventions following the Geneva Convention of 1925 established and extended an import certificate system together with limitation of manufacture. A separate opium section of the League of Nations was created in 1930.

The key international developments in public health in the interwar years, corporate philanthropy and the League of Nations, were closely connected. The LNHO drew between a third and a half of its health budget from the Rockefeller Foundation. The foundation helped Ludwik Rajchman, the League of Nation's medical director, to recruit staff, gave travel grants allowing individuals to visit Geneva, recommended members of expert bodies, made its own staff available for special purposes, and helped assess requests for technical assistance. Such linkages again are relevant to consideration of the contemporary role of corporate philanthropy and public–private partnerships in international health and its organizations, which have been long-lasting.

International health after World War II

The LNHO survived World War II and was present at the first World Health Assembly (WHA) held in Geneva in 1948. It subsequently merged with UNRRA, the United Nations Relief and Rehabilitation Administration, founded to deal with the relief and repatriation of refugees in Europe after the war, and the Office Internationale D'Hygiene Publique, to form the core of the new WHO which emerged from the WHA.

Public health became a European concept through the post-war refugee crisis. The Soviet Union and other communist states were not involved in the WHO between 1949 and 1956, but the United States was—the first time it had joined such an international organization. This country balance ensured that the focus of the new organization was on technical interventions aimed at improving medical capacity and health planning in member countries, but it excluded direct funding of health infrastructure. Its technical assistance model marked a retreat from its roots in social medicine ideas, although these had become associated with narrower laboratory-based approaches before the war. UNICEF, the new UN children's organization, was also closely involved in health, its target group including both mothers and children.

One of the earliest programmes supported and initiated by the WHO and donor agencies was against malaria. The war had drawn attention to the powerful influence of the disease, which had caused more casualties among the troops in Asia and the Pacific areas than the war itself. The WHO malaria eradication programme was launched in 1955, based on the twin-pronged attack of DDT against the vector and chloroquine as a human prophylaxis (Figure 9).

Earlier, before the war, malariologists had debated different approaches to eradication. Vertical programmes would eliminate the mosquito through draining, oiling, and employing 'mosquito brigades' to patrol the sites. A healthier workforce would then

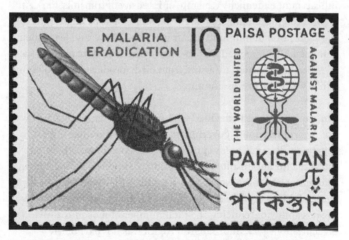

9. Campaigns against malaria were initiated by the newly formed WHO in the 1950s. High-tech solutions were in favour in medicine and public health in this decade, and DDT was widely used; spraying was later curtailed because of growing fears about the environmental impact.

achieve economic development. Other malariologists supported a horizontal programme. The decline of malaria in Europe before the war suggested that if a reasonable standard of living, employment, economic development, and education were in place then malaria would fade out as a consequence. This horizontal/vertical divide and its assumptions prefigured many of the later debates surrounding public health strategies at international and national levels.

After the war, technical solutions came to the fore with the advent of DDT. First synthesized in 1874, it was originally designed not for malaria, but for typhus. Research awarded the Nobel Prize in 1948 transformed the pesticide into a powerful residual insecticide. Rockefeller-funded malaria eradication campaigns under the direction of Fred Soper in Egypt and Sardinia drove enthusiasm for scaling up DDT into a global eradication programme. Researchers in Africa were wary of an eradication programme that did not take into account endemicity (the rate or intensity of transmission). An eradication programme in a high-transmission area might interrupt the acquisition of immunity of African populations and leave them vulnerable. They argued that the high rates of malaria in some parts of Africa, the constant exposure from birth, produced a population which was more or less immune.

The campaign was bedevilled with problems from the start. It was not incorporated into government health programmes but sat separately. In some areas spraying was needed more often than budgeted for and resulted in depletion of supplies. The results in different parts of the world were variable—they were more successful in economically developed states or on islands where the possibility of reducing the total number of mosquitos was an achievable goal. Sub-Saharan Africa was not part of the programme but was the area with the greatest disease challenge. A growing environmental movement stimulated by Rachel Carson and her book, *Silent Spring* (1962), criticized the use of DDT as a poison and possible carcinogen with long-term effects.

In 1969 the malaria programme was converted, with less publicity, to a focus on control.

The programme had epitomized the post-war optimism about health and the faith in technical solutions which animated much of the work of the WHO in the 1950s. A global yaws campaign from 1952 to 1964 treated upwards of fifty million people with one injection of long-acting penicillin. The much less high-profile area of alcohol, previously the province of temperance rather than public health, achieved considerable attention with a focus on the idea of 'disease' and the provision of specialists to treat alcoholism. The WHO's work in mental health more generally underlined the inclusion of this area within the ambit of public health.

The optimism of the post-war programmes depended crucially on new antibiotics and pesticides. Penicillin and related antibiotics and sulphonamide drugs were widely trialled in these programmes. The smallpox eradication campaign (1967–79) was hailed as a success. The last naturally occurring case was in 1977 and the disease was ratified as extinct in human populations in 1980. Bynum points out that it was less a triumph of medical science and more one for vaccination, and long-established public health methods of case tracking, isolation, and mass vaccination of populations at risk. In parts of South East Asia, its final stages in 1973–5 were marked by intimidation of local health officials and coercive vaccination. It was essentially an administrative campaign.

The rise of primary health care and health promotion

The technical focus of the immediate post-war period at the international level was also marked in the way health systems were established in developing countries, many achieving independence in this period. Health budgets went towards teaching hospitals, importing diagnostic and therapeutic technology, and costly medicines. By the 1970s there was a reaction against the importation of Western or industrialized models of health care. This chimed with developments in the West, where high-tech medicine and the impact of public health were also being increasingly criticized. We saw in Chapter 5 how the McKeown thesis used historical data to argue for the greater influence of nutritional and living standards on health; and writers such as Ivan Illich and Thomas Szasz also argued against the dominance of medicine. The rising costs of health care and the impact of oil price rises, imposed by the Organization of Petroleum Exporting Countries at the end of 1973, had major consequences for Western economies and limited what could be spent on health services.

Alternative ways of developing health care and public health came on to the agenda. In developing countries the primary health care movement was of great importance, while in the developed world a new version of public health—called health promotion—came into being. Both were international movements. Primary health care was different from health promotion because it focused to a greater extent on the treatment of disease and on services.

Maurice King's *Medical Care in Developing Countries* (1966) became the bible for English-speaking health workers in these countries. Health services were attempting to treat diseases which could have been prevented. The underlying cause of much disease was poverty and so solutions other than technical medical ones had to be sought. King advocated moving health services closer to the populations they served and using medical auxiliaries rather than fully trained doctors. Such ideas were implemented in the late 1960s in Tanzania, and the idea of prevention was given greater emphasis.

In China too there were alternatives to existing health services, and the system of barefoot doctors came into existence after the cultural revolution of 1966–9 had shifted attention to rural areas.

Barefoot doctors were health workers who did that work in their time off from labouring in the fields. Although China was at this stage a low income country, life expectancy improved from 47 years in 1960 to 67 years in 1980, and preventive programmes greatly decreased the prevalence of diseases such as schistosomiasis (bilharzia). Venezuela, Guatemala, Costa Rica, and Cuba, which had lost one-third of its doctors after the revolution, developed similar models.

Such ideas seeped into the WHO and helped to define the primary health care approach. The failure of the malaria eradication programme as a vertical programme also influenced new directions. Throughout the 1970s the WHO worked on studying alternatives, and the organization itself began to take a much more active role in persuasion and promotion of a particular health message. This change of stance was led by Halfdan Mahler, who became director-general in 1973. In 1975, he launched the idea of 'Health for All by the Year 2000' as WHO's contribution to the UN 'New International Economic Order'. Health had to be considered as part of the contribution to social development. Such was the context of ideas when the International Conference on Primary Health Care was held at Alma Ata in 1978. It was sponsored by WHO and UNICEF with a substantial financial contribution from the host country, the Soviet Union. The declaration of Alma Ata outlined the role of primary health care (PHC) in the aim of Health for All by the Year 2000 (HFA).

The main elements of PHC at Alma Ata comprised elements of what we might consider a public health approach—proper food and nutrition; safe water and basic sanitation; education on health problems and their prevention; maternal and child health including family planning; immunization; prevention of locally endemic diseases; as well as treatment and provision of essential drugs. It was the first example of target-setting at the international level, a strategy replicated since in the Millennium Development Goals. But in the years after Alma Ata, the PHC approach became mired in disputes and debates between proponents of different ways of achieving its goals. These crystallized as a debate between universal and selective PHC.

Should primary care be a vertical or a horizontal movement? What vertical meant in this case was a narrowing focus on particular conditions or groups rather than the broader approach originally envisaged. The historian Marcos Cueto has commented that this meant a package of low-cost technical interventions to tackle the main disease problems of poor countries. The package was known as GOBI, comprising four main interventions: growth monitoring, oral rehydration techniques, breast feeding, and immunization. These were easy to monitor and attracted the support of UNICEF, which stressed the need to do the best with finite resources and with political opportunities. This narrower focus was also tied into the priorities of international health donors who wanted to fund these initiatives.

The health promotion movement was different, although it was also influenced by the need to move away from reliance on formal and high-tech health systems. Health promotion emerged during the 1970s and 1980s with a 'Canadian–European' focus. Canadian initiatives in public health were important, in particular the publication in 1974 of the Lalonde Report, *A New Perspective on the Health of Canadians*. Lalonde, who was Canadian Minister of Health, stressed the non-medical approach and the inadequacies of PHC provision, emphasizing the role of social structures in promoting health. Behaviour was important, as in lifestyle public health, but this was behaviour at both individual and corporate levels.

Individual countries produced policy documents based on this ideal—*Prevention and Health: Everybody's Business* in the UK in 1976, for example. The work of the WHO and its regional offices was important in taking this ideal forward. The Pan American Health Organization and WHO's European regional office (WHO EURO) played key roles. In 1984 WHO EURO adopted thirty-eight targets to achieve the HFA goal. The WHO regional committee took the line that lifestyles needed to be understood as collective behaviours rooted in social context. The approach gave public health a focus on social reform and equity. In 1986, at a conference held in Ottawa, Canada, under the leadership of WHO and Mahler, the Ottawa Charter for Health Promotion was adopted. This moved the focus of public health from disease prevention to 'capacity building for health'. It stated:

> The fundamental conditions and resources for health are peace, shelter, education, income, a stable ecosystem, sustainable resources, social justice and equity. Improvement in health requires a secure foundation in these basic prerequisites.

In some countries, such as the US, health promotion remained more closely tied to health education and chronic disease prevention (because of the longer history of the concept of chronic disease in the US). But WHO EURO and its Health Education Unit, led by the sociologist Ilona Kickbusch, developed the 'settings' approach, which focused on creating networks.

The regional office began to work with local authorities, cities, universities, organizations, hospitals, and schools. In 1987, the Healthy Cities initiative was launched. This explicitly bypassed national ministries and aimed to localize health promotion with a strong lobby at that level. In Liverpool in England, a regional health promotion group developed in the local Mersey Regional Health Authority, and Howard Seymour became the country's first Regional Health Promotion Officer. Health promotion was in an uneasy relationship and often in opposition to another development called 'new public health', which attempted to define health promotion as a subset of its activities. Some argued that this was a tactic to regain the initiative for medical public health interests from health promotion, whose workers were multidisciplinary and not exclusively medical. In the UK, the subsequent rise of multidisciplinary public health and the change from public health as a medical-only occupation built on both health promotion and new public health.

The 1970s had seen the elaboration of a standard 'public health package' of measures which public health aimed for at the national level in the UK, among them a new hostility to industrial interests which replaced the previous cooperation in a shared agenda. Hostility also marked activities on the international scene. Tension between industrial interests and health activist groups (here characterized as NGOs) began to emerge at this time. The attack on the marketing policies of transnational corporations such as Nestlé was part of this new direction for international public health. In 1981, amid protest from the US government and transnational corporations, the WHA adopted an International Code for the Marketing of Breast Milk Substitutes. This was the culmination of international protest on the issue, following an earlier WHA resolution in 1974 and the call in 1977 for a boycott of Nestlé products by the Infant Formula Action Coalition. Activists were concerned that expensive and sometimes insanitary bottle-feeding was being promoted for commercial reasons to the detriment of breast feeding. The ability to develop a consumer boycott of a global product range on a health and development issue was new.

The 1980s: structural adjustment and HIV/AIDS

PHC and health promotion/new public health were not the only movements on the international health agenda. Population growth and nutrition were also areas of concern. Since the 1960s there had been fears that the world's resources were finite and that pollution, misuse of existing resources, and consumption demands were all increasing.

The World Bank and its president, the American Robert McNamara, focused on the 'population explosion' in the late 1970s and 1980s, and large amounts of money were spent on population control activities by international donors. The financial crisis of the 1970s brought a new donor-driven approach to countries in the global South. The large-scale introduction of International Monetary Fund-sponsored 'structural adjustment programmes' brought the decline of state-run public health programmes and the return of the diseases of poverty and also infectious disease. The neo-liberal 1980s saw mandatory privatization of utilities such as water supplies and the handing over of control to multinational companies.

In the midst of this deterioration in public health structures and capacity came a new epidemic: HIV/AIDS. The initial presentation of the disease as an 'old disease from Africa' had clear resonances with earlier racialized discourses on STDs. The perception of HIV as an African crisis also led to moves to understand its spread there. Historical demographers working on Africa concluded that the 'prehistory' of the growth of urban centres, and the rise in unemployment and female poverty after the 1973 oil crisis, had helped pave the way for the epidemic spread of the disease. The responses at a country level in Africa differed, with a policy based on abstinence in Uganda in contrast to one based on rejection of Western biomedicine in South Africa under president Thabo Mbeki. AIDS was more than an African problem, and by the turn of the 21st century one-quarter of people with AIDS were in Asia, especially India. AIDS was also a global problem, and in 1986 the WHO established a Global Programme on AIDS, which began to fund AIDS programmes in low and middle income countries. AIDS was a harbinger of the new focus on globalism in health; the human rights discourse which had animated programmes in the global North also transferred into countries of the global South.

So from the 19th century through to the 20th century, public health moved from imperial to global health. Tropical medicine had been inspired by European needs and colonial strategies. A different world emerged after World War II, with new international movements and variants of public health located in a expanding range of international and global institutions.

Chapter 7
Present and future in the light of history

In 2015, the *Lancet* held a competition and subsequently published some views from its readers about the health of the UK population in 2040. One contribution, written by a public health academic from Liverpool University, presented a dystopian cautionary science-fiction tale:

I live in a city with harsh winters and savage hurricanes in summers. I supplement my income by wearing smart contact lenses, that paid me pennies for watching adverts. This kept me away from the outsourced social police. Diabetes is everywhere and helping tuberculosis to bite again angrily in our cities. Diseases like Ebola are still there, still waiting for a vaccine and still neglected, at least when contained somewhere in Africa. Famines are happening even at home: Many of us can just afford simple healthy food, despite our technical abilities to convert soya beans in whatever way we want.... Battles that my dad told me that were almost 'won' are now lost, like new old ways of maximising profits by delivering known harmful substances ..not surprisingly, cardiovascular disease started to rise again, particularly amongst the poorest of us Just a few years after they stopped negotiating in 2016, a century of continued decline in deaths was reversed. Sad, but profitable to those selling cheap DIY coronary artery disease stem-cell repair kits in Lime Street station vending machines.

We saw this coming in 2015: We've lost the battle to tame
corporations.

The contribution was tongue in cheek and painted a disturbing
picture of what the future of the health of the public might be.
Present and future possibilities are the subject of this final
chapter. The *Lancet* competition fed into an enquiry by the
prestigious British Academy of Medical Sciences about what the
health of the public might look like in 2040. This enquiry pointed
out that there had been changes for the better in public health and
changes for the worse over the previous fifty years. Life expectancy
had increased in the UK. Reduced rates of smoking had played a
part there as well as improvements in nutrition, work patterns, air
quality, hygiene, and biomedical interventions. Health protection
had also brought improvement with fewer traffic fatalities because
of seatbelt and drink driving laws. Women's health had improved
with safe contraception, abortion, and childbirth. Attitudes
towards sexuality, personal responsibility, and mental health
had all changed with a better-educated public that was more
health literate.

Other changes had brought the opposite effect, particularly with
regard to the rise of non-communicable diseases. Sedentary
lifestyles, the impact of sugar, fast food, and marketing on
diets had brought problems with obesity. Stressful lifestyles
brought worsening mental health. There were continuing social
inequalities both in life expectancy and patterns of health
behaviour, and while life expectancy had increased across all
socio-economic strata, inequalities between them had
persisted. Attitudes towards vaccination on the part of the
public remained wary, compromised by uncertain science and
decreasing awareness of the diseases vaccination prevented.
The environment had changed for the better overall, but health
outcomes might be increasingly shaped by environmental
degradation, pollution, and rising consumption of both energy
and processed foods.

Any future scenario is likely to be swiftly overtaken by events. It is possible to outline some possibilities and emergent as well as long-standing issues. The recent histories of public health at the national and international levels ended with a similar development – the revival of infectious disease and in particular the arrival of HIV/AIDS. In recent decades there has been a growing commonality between North and South, or between high, middle, and low income countries. One feature of the future scenario is likely to be increased interdependence between issues at the national and at the international or global levels, and so here both are discussed together.

Definitions of public health

At the start of this book I outlined a series of changing and time-dependent definitions for public health; and noted that public health was amorphous, defining itself around whatever activities it undertook at a particular point in time. This indeterminate nature is unlikely to change: what counts as public health and what is emphasized will continue to vary depending on external factors and circumstances and who, and which, institutions and groups are involved. It had been predicted that by 2020 the term public health would no longer be used. Instead the terms would be 'health improvement and well-being'. As we have seen, there have been a multitude of terms used over time and there will be more in the future. But the public recognizes the term 'public health'—even if they are not always sure what it means –and so it is likely to stay in use.

Earlier chapters outlined a series of stages whereby a focus on the environment and on sanitation in the 19th century gave way under the impact of scientific advance, germ theory in particular, to a greater emphasis on the role of the individual and in particular individual mothers. Post-World War II, that focus on the individual was maintained, although in a different way with different, chronic, or non-communicable conditions in view, through the focus on the modification of individual behaviour and of lifestyle, but always in the context of the epidemiological role of the whole population. Recently, there has been a revival of the environmental focus of the 19th century, but this time with the global environment as the concern, with new public health issues such as transport on the agenda. Early 21st-century public health combines both an individual behavioural and an environmental population focus. The sustainable development and public health agendas are coming together. In what follows, using the headings first used in Chapter 2, we will look at how some of these issues may pan out.

Topics and tactics

Changes in the natural environment span countries in the North and South. The potential to reduce carbon emissions and meet water efficiency and reduction targets is likely to be key to health. There could be changes in agriculture, the state of ecosystems, and the availability of food, energy, and water. Energy deficits and changes in migration may come into play and coincide with increasing climate stresses.

The post-war trend was the rise of lifestyle-related conditions as central to public health and the decline of infectious diseases. But will those trends be maintained? Will public health will be focusing on *non-communicable diseases* (NCDs), the major issue of the post-World War II decades, or will there will be a *continued revival of infectious disease and viral pandemics*?

This dichotomy affects high, middle, and low income countries. In the low and middle income countries the arrival of chronic NCDs has recently emerged as a key issue. Over the last ten years, there has been mounting alarm about the growth of NCDs there. These have been defined as four conditions (cardiovascular disease, cancer, diabetes, and chronic respiratory disorders), related to four behavioural risk factors (diet, physical activity, smoking, and alcohol). More than 60 per cent of deaths worldwide were attributed to NCDs, and nearly 80 per cent of these deaths occurred in low and middle income countries. They were the negative consequence of socio-economic development, with economic growth and rapid urbanization bringing in their train modern lifestyles like smoking and drinking. International organizations such as the WHO have published reports and action plans, and a Political Declaration on the Prevention and Control of NCDs was passed at the United Nations.

At the same time, infectious diseases pose a new threat both nationally and also globally. HIV/AIDS in the 1980s presaged a new role for infectious disease in public health. In 2014, Ebola, first identified in 1976, became an epidemic in West Africa: in Guinea, Liberia, and Sierra Leone. More than 800 health care workers contracted the disease and 500 died. The epidemic attracted input from experienced overseas NGOs like Médecins Sans Frontières, and infected health care workers were flown back to be treated in the very different health care systems of their home countries. Old fears of the arrival of infectious disease from far distant countries were aroused. Ebola did not spread in the UK as cholera had done in the 19th century. Border controls were put in place by the government; these were widely criticized as unnecessary and ineffective. The epidemic raised many issues in relation to public health systems at the country level and also globally. Increasing globalization, the increasing flow of people from place to place, and changing climactic conditions could potentially increase the risk from new and emerging infectious diseases such as Ebola and also from novel respiratory infections (Figure 10).

How governments responded was always a fine balance of risk. In 2009, when swine flu (H1N1) arrived in the UK, public health authorities and the government reacted with a high-level emergency response, the opening of special flu centres, and the purchase of large amounts of vaccine. This was subsequently

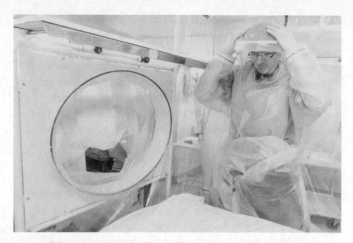

10. Health care workers dealing with the Ebola epidemic in 2014. The outbreaks of Ebola in West Africa in 2014 highlighted many public health issues: the globalization of infectious disease; criticism of the role of the WHO in responding to the epidemic; the importance of understanding local beliefs in fighting disease; and the wider issue of strengthening local health systems rather than simply dealing with the immediate emergency.

criticized as an overreaction and the WHO was criticized for doing too much. Peter Piot, one of the first people to work on the Ebola virus in the 1970s and later head of UNAIDS, remarked, 'We don't know at the beginning of an epidemic how it will pan out...we will have to overreach and not take the risk.' Such calculations of risk about the national and global spread of infectious disease are likely to be the case in the future. Concerns about re-emergent infectious disease also focus on biosecurity. As well as pandemic flu and other epidemics, there is a greater possibility of chemical, biological, radiological, or nuclear release, possibly linked to the global impact of wars and terrorism. The 21st century has so far been an era of migration and this has brought public health issues such as sanitation and epidemic disease spread in its train, with parallels to the refugee crisis in Europe after World War II.

Changing behaviours will still be central to public health in the future. Behaviours are increasingly seen in their environmental, economic, and social context. The power of vested interests, combined with the role of individual responsibility and personal behaviour change, presents a future challenge. The agency Public Health England, in evidence to the Academy of Medical Science enquiry, talked of 'the increasingly obesogenic, polluted and populated environment' which would require complex and population based interventions.

Ideas about individual behaviour change are now related to the environment in which the individual made those decisions. For obesity for example, this involves the role of the food industry—issues such as labelling and information, but also the wider environment in terms how available cheaper food is, the policies adopted by supermarkets, the positioning of local shops, and planning decisions made by councils about the location and accessibility of food outlets. Individual behaviour is still part of the issue, with advice about exercise and healthy eating. But a public health response could also involve surgical intervention. The growing availability of bariatric surgery for obesity underlines the blurred boundary between public health and clinical approaches—the relationship of public health with health services. The definition of overeating as a 'brain disease' with people needing their sugar 'fix' demonstrates the expansion of neuroscientific models into public health. Calls for a sugar tax, however, underline the continuation of traditional public health calls for taxation of unhealthy products. In 2015, the WHO published a report drawing parallels with smoking. Public health strategies are variable and also dependent on national location: the brain science model has had more purchase in the US.

Obesity is a key issue on the future behavioural agenda, as is alcohol consumption. Illicit drugs have come into the public health field in the wake of HIV/AIDS but the salience of drugs within public health is changing. The boundaries between legal and illegal substances are more porous than previously, as is the boundary between medical and non-medical usage. Smart drugs and legal highs pose new conundrums for control, but also demonstrate the spread of drug use more widely in society and the greater acceptability of enhancing performance through using drugs.

Smoking, the classic post-war public health behavioural issue, is less important than it had been in the UK, and public health campaigners are concerned about how to keep it in view on the public health agenda. The future of harm reduction remains in doubt as e-cigarette consumption plateaus. How such products are to be regulated varies by country and also at the European level. In the United States, there is confusion about whether they count as 'tobacco products' and could therefore be regulated by the Food and Drug Administration under the 2009 Family Smoking Prevention and Tobacco Control Act. In low and middle income countries, however, smoking and the role of 'big tobacco' remains an important issue. Public health campaigners have drawn attention to the way in which the tobacco industry had shifted its attention to low and middle income countries where controls were limited. But restrictions on smoking put in place in China in 2015 presaged new attitudes to control and health in one of the major world smoking markets.

The cross-cutting issue of inequality will remain important in the future. No longer, as in the 1980s, is it a topic which could not be mentioned. But the health of the public continues to be influenced by socio-economic, gender, and other forms of inequality, as well as housing and the effects of class and location on access to and quality of health services. In the medium term, differential access to technology and heath related resources is likely to be a key influencing factor, along with the extent to which the wealthy lose or gain influence and there is a more or less equitable distribution of health and resources.

What about tactics?

The rise of *antimicrobial resistance* threatens some of the gains made by public health. Tuberculosis is making a comeback despite the introduction of directly observed therapy, a widely used tactic for ensuring that treatment regimes are completed in order to increase compliance. The overuse of antibiotics to promote growth and productivity in animals as well as their use in humans threatens to increase antibiotic resistance in both humans and animals—an example of the increased entwining of human and animal public health issues since BSE. This gives added weight to arguments for vaccination as a tactic both nationally and as central to programmes in low and middle income countries.

Public health genomics and screening is another area of increased salience on the public health agenda. The mapping of the human genome gives greater potential for identifying relationships between genes and diseases. The prospect has been raised of further genetic testing of those at risk of particular diseases as well as population-wide programmes. The possibility could develop of screening programmes which profile an individual's risk of developing cancer or heart disease. Genetic screening might reassure people that their risks are low, reducing anxiety. People at higher risk might benefit from increased surveillance and earlier intervention. The impact on lifestyle is debated. Would low-risk individuals reject healthy living, believing they were invincible? Would high-risk individuals adopt a fatalistic approach? Should people be told—do they want to know?

A range of harms is sometimes associated with screening, such as heightened anxiety and unnecessary treatment. Radical treatment might be carried out—mastectomy for early breast cancer for example—even though it is not certain the disease would develop. Genetic screening also carries a range of adverse social implications. Those at risk can be discriminated against—by employers or by banks and insurance companies. There are issues of confidentiality—how will the information be handled and who will access test results? The emphasis on genetic screening could shift attention away from other causes of disease, associated with lifestyle and environmental factors. The enthusiasm in some quarters for the genetic approach recalls public health's focus at the turn of the 19th and 20th centuries when explanations of disease were in terms of heredity, although of course the remedies proposed in the present are different. Genetic screening and targeted treatments also raise the issue of the resources available in countries and who is able to afford them. Increasing cost and specialized knowledge is a threat to equity and access.

The *rise of explanations based on neuroscience* is also redolent with history—the 19th-century interest in the brain in terms of the location of different diseases and also the ways in which brain science had been linked to degenerationist theories at the turn of the 19th and 20th centuries. Scientists in the US argue that addiction is a chronic relapsing brain disease and this has brought greater emphasis on drug treatment and the role of pharmaceuticals rather than environmental or lifestyle change or concern about the role of poverty and inequality. Expansion of the brain science model has begun to encompass other lifestyle activities such as eating, sex, and gambling. This accommodation of public health lifestyle perspectives and brain science is a stronger trend in the US than in Europe, driven in part by scientific traditions with their genetic focus and also by the needs of an insurance-driven health care system. To hear a leading neuroscientist talk of success in manipulating the brains of drug users as a treatment option brings shadows of the eugenic past.

Public health ethics

Genetics emphasize another development in public health—the rise of a distinctive public health ethics, separate from more general ethical concerns in medicine. Ethical dilemmas in public health practice are given greater attention. To some degree this spills over from the health promotion field in public health where the application of ethical principles such as 'to do no harm' have long been applied as a test of interventions.

In 2007, the UK Nuffield Council on Bioethics reported on ethical issues in public health. It adopted a revised liberal framework based on the notion of stewardship, that liberal states had responsibilities for the needs of people both individually and collectively. States should be interventionist in public health matters but not coercive unless there was an extreme threat. Public health programmes should reduce the risks of ill health which people might impose on each other; ensure environmental conditions that sustain good health; pay special attention to vulnerable groups such as children; provide information and advice for people to overcome unhealthy behaviours; reduce unfair health inequalities; and so on. Coercion into leading healthy lives was ruled out, and interventions should not be introduced without consent or adequate mandate. The Council also identified third parties with an important role in public health. These included publicly funded bodies and charities, and also business organizations. In situations of market failure or where business did not act responsibly, then governments could intervene. The rise of an interest in human rights in public health was also part of this ethical concern.

Education and the rise of social media and new technology

Education, as earlier chapters have shown, had long been a key public health tactic. Here new technology brought fresh challenges, both for self-education and for educating 'the public' as a whole. Schools and workplaces are seen as key sites. Increasing emphases on social networks, health tracking, and self-measurement provide new means to alter behaviour but are also complicated by issues of data ownership, privacy, and interoperability. The uneven adoption of new technology at the individual level also presents the risk of a digital divide on the basis of age and socio-economic status. In terms of education of the public, new possibilities have emerged. The industry approach has moved away from a whole population approach for advertising towards targeting individuals, groups, and age groups through social media. Public health tactics operate in a similar way.

The targeted groups

Public health continues its traditional focus on young age groups: the health and well-being of children and young people remains a key concern. But the public health implications of an ageing population have increasingly come to the fore. In a survey of leading public health practitioners in 2007, this emergent problem recurred again and again. One contributor commented that the key public health question for the next ten or twenty years would be how to address the health and care needs of a growing elderly population, and in particular how that care would be funded. Another predicted that ageing populations combined with obesity would drive increases in long-term conditions: these could be cured but would require the promotion of healthy active lifestyles. The ageing population was also associated with the rise in mental health problems and dementia.

Historians have critiqued the continuing public health focus on the 'future of the race' in terms of women, mothers, and children. Men tend to be ignored even when, as with drinking, they are a major part of the problem. Historical research also casts doubt on some of the arguments about the 'problem' of the elderly. This fear of the elderly had emerged at other points in history and was rarely justified by events. The increasing numbers of active elderly and their community contribution has been disregarded. Women up to the age of 75, for example, give the community more than they take in terms of services. The 'problem' argument fails to distinguish between the different stages of old age and their public health implications.

Institutions and locations

The institutions and locations of public health will not remain unchanged. At the global level, the role of the WHO has come in for criticism because of its fragmented response to the Ebola epidemic. The director-general of the organization, Margaret Chan, defending its record in a speech at the London School of Hygiene and Tropical Medicine in 2015, admitted that the WHO had underestimated the situation. The disease had crossed borders and there was reinfection. Cultural traditions of caring for the diseased and dying mitigated against containment, and health messages backfired. Families preferred to rely on traditional healers and care for patients at home. But there were also wider issues. Critics pointed out that the WHO had disbanded its early rapid response team and failed to check the progress of the disease in Guinea early in 2014.

Ebola also raised other issues—the failure to adopt international health regulations and the way in which external global funds had skewed health funding in the affected countries and had created dependence. External public health funding had focused on particular diseases and had not strengthened health systems. Surveillance and laboratory systems needed to be in place, but only sixty-four countries within the WHO (one-third of its total membership) had such facilities. The role of anthropology as a public health research tool was promoted because it had enabled local attitudes to be understood. The basics of establishing a public health response were lacking and greater emphasis needed to be placed, so it was argued, on sustainable development. Vertical systems were not the only way to go. One commentator spoke of how the smallpox external funding had left behind 'graveyards of vehicles which were not maintained' and this had done little to create the systems which were really needed.

Better leadership from the WHO was being called for, but the dispersal of power at the international level through private foundations and other global institutions seems likely to continue. The health-related MDGs had led to a disease-focused organization, the Global Fund. The goals had not been met by the time the United Nations final report was published in 2015. The eight goals—on poverty, education, gender equality, child mortality, maternal health, disease, the environment, and global partnership, had yielded mixed results. The target for tackling malaria had been achieved, due to a tenfold increase in international financing since 2000 and sustained prevention and treatment. The global malaria incidence rate had fallen by more than a third and the mortality rate by more than a half. But those in the development field point out that technological advances alone will not work without improvements in health systems and reduction of inequities. That, and improved social and political governance, is fundamental to the basis of malaria control before elimination can even be thought of. The target of halving the proportion of people without access to improved sources of water was achieved in 2010. In 2015 a new set of targets, the Sustainable Development Goals, were put in place for fifteen years as successors to the MDGs.

The expansion of global organizations impacting on public health continues. The WTO, for example, with its role in the protection and enforcement of trade-related intellectual property rights (TRIPS), remains contentious as far as health is concerned. Commentators draw attention to the way in which TRIPS are used by the tobacco industry to counter the restrictions on advertising, promotion, and smuggling of tobacco imposed by the Framework Convention on Tobacco Control, which arguably impose a barrier to free trade. The general response of the WTO governing bodies when health and free trade came into conflict, is to defer responsibility to the national level.

Europe seems likely to continue and to expand its activity in public health. Its powers could be extended through the back door in the form of regulations in areas such as health and safety, food standards, trade, and the environment, and through its social policy programmes. WHO EURO, which had lost ground in relation to the EU, also seems to be developing a new public health role with its blueprint Health 2020.

Within the UK, the impact of devolution will continue to impact on public health provision, as Scotland and England already have distinctively different health service structures. Historically Scotland had also developed different public health strategies, often pioneering approaches which were later taken up further south. It pioneered 'harm reduction' for injecting drug use in the wake of HIV/AIDS, and some of the early anti-tobacco advertising strategies—gaining the support of the Scotland football team for example—were first used in Scotland and then transferred into England. The latest example of this creative tension between the two countries is the issue of minimum unit pricing for alcohol, where the Scottish parliament took the lead but its decision was under legal challenge by the Scotch Whisky Association. In Northern Ireland there is more joint working with public health in the south to tackle issues on an all Ireland basis.

Diversity and devolution is also the case in England with public health's move into local government. The focus on localism has made spatial unevenness and different provision a distinct possibility. Public health budgets have initially been ring-fenced, with an increase in funding for local authorities with the worst socio-economic conditions. Removal of ring-fencing has given councils flexibility in mitigating local government budget cuts from central government, but the danger might be that public health funds become dissipated by other local government priorities. For drug and alcohol treatment, large voluntary-sector providers have been awarded contracts, and specialist services are under threat. Research evidence on the impact of the move to local government is thin on the ground, but there is evidence, in

117

an era of central government cuts, that making savings is an important criterion for politicians.

The national role of public health is represented by the CMO's role in government and also by the agency Public Health England. The response to swine flu in 2009 had shown tensions between different approaches to risk communication on the part of the CMO Sir Liam Donaldson and public health, as represented in the Health Protection Agency (HPA). At the local level, too, there has been confusion between the public health responses from the HPA, the NHS, and local government agencies. Reorganization meant that some of these issues are framed differently. Public Health England is less independent of government than the HPA had been, an issue which caused concern at the time of reorganization. It was argued too that its connections and ability to influence the local level were attenuated and weak.

Public health people

The public health workforce in England has mostly moved out of the NHS and into local government, and its multidisciplinarity has also expanded. There has been the challenge of developing relationships across a range of local government directorates from housing, planning, and transport, to alcohol licensing. People who work in those areas and in the voluntary sector can also be seen as part of the public health workforce. Some argue that the specialist public health function is in decline except in certain areas such as health protection. Training, too, is under discussion. Academic public health training tends to focus on technocratic skills such as epidemiology and statistics. But in the political context of local government there is less reverence for 'the evidence' and better communication and political/negotiating skills might be necessary. Earlier MoHs had known this well. Paddy Donaldson, the father of the former CMO, Sir Liam Donaldson, had operated shrewdly in the context of Stockton on Tees in the 1960s and, before him, Arthur Newsholme had used the local political context to achieve public health aims when he was MoH in Brighton in the 1900s. At the national level, one commentator pointed out that in 2015, neither the CMO nor the head of Public Health England had public health training.

Critiques of public health

What about critiques of public health? The tension between technical fix and overarching vision is still current, nowhere more so than in the global health field where it was highlighted by responses to the Ebola epidemic. Vaccination as a tactic still epitomizes the tension between the individual and the collective benefit. The 'nanny state' argument is less often advanced than it had been, although it is still around. Times have changed; and health campaigns are no longer just the responsibility of government departments, but often run by other interests. Drinkaware, funded at arm's length by the alcohol industry, is running public health campaigns about alcohol. Self-awareness and self-monitoring (blood pressure monitors, pedometers, and the like) have become lucrative businesses. The blurring of boundaries between clinical or surgical intervention, drug treatment, and behavioural strategies (as in the field of obesity) have taken some of the force away from the 'nanny state' critique. Multi-drug resistance for infectious disease is another example of the interlinking of public health and medicine. The revival of infectious disease and its global impact has brought issues of over- or underreaction by public health interests more to the fore.

The present and future in the light of the past promotes reflection. History is ongoing and teaches us about change. It cannot be assumed that the present state of play in public health will always be the same. Public health in the past moved through distinct stages as the chapters of this book have outlined. The latest stage is the outgrowth of those earlier ones and defined by the structures and imperatives of the present. One can see in the present how environmental ideas, reformulated from the 19th-century concern for sanitation to encompass climate change, have come back into public health.

At the same time, the post-World War II reorientation of public health towards lifestyle and the population has taken on a new dimension as drug treatments and brain science also move into the public health arena. A pharmaceutical public health is part of the current 21st-century picture, epitomized by the rise of pre-exposure prophylaxis for HIV/AIDS (PrEP). The tension between the individual in public health and the population has taken on new dimensions, although with resonance with the past. The standard public health package of high taxation, focus on the media, and opposition to industry was established in the 1970s. But is that automatic response changing? The mass media are in decline, and could industry (for example the pharmaceutical industry) be part of the solution to public health problems?

Public health will always be the 'art of the possible' and its amoeba-like compass remains—embracing health services and medication (as with statins); the environment and transport; brain science; and lifestyle. It is related to country structures and systems and to whether the state is a centralized one (as in England) or whether there is a Federal/state divide (as in the US and Australia for example). Types of international agencies and private philanthropy may have changed over time, but distinct continuities are there between pre- and post-World War II international and global health. The focus of public health—blaming women for example, talking about the 'innocent victims', the concern for children and young people, the 'future of the race'—remains constant.

Looking at the history of public health does not offer policy prescriptions for the future, but it can create greater awareness of the determinants of the present. In Chapter 1, we discussed how the standard critiques of public health were in contrast with the enthusiasm and advocacy which characterized the public health field. Using history to understand the present helps potentially to bring those diverse strands together.

References

Chapter 1: What is public health?

C. E. A. Winslow's definition of public health is in 'The Untilled Fields of Public Health', *Science*, 51 (1920): 23. The WHO definition of health is from the organization's founding constitution of 1948. The 1988 definition is taken from the Acheson Report, *Public Health in England. The Report of the Committee of Inquiry into the future development of the public health function* (London: Department of Health, 1988). The Wanless Report definition is in *Securing Good Health for the Whole Population* (London: HMSO, 2004), p. 27.

Chapter 2: Current challenges

The Faculty of Public Health priorities are taken from my notes of the annual meeting in 2014.

The comments about 'nudge' and 'shove' were made by Professor David Hunter.

Chapter 3: The origins of public health into the 1700s

Rosen's comment is from *A History of Public Health*, expanded edition with introduction by Elizabeth Fee (Baltimore, MD: Johns Hopkins University Press, 1993), p. 29.

Chapter 4: Sanitation to education: 1800–1900s

Christopher Hamlin's critique of public health comes from *Public Health and Social Justice in the Age of Chadwick: Britain, 1800–1854* (Cambridge: Cambridge University Press, 1998), p. 12.

Chapter 5: The rise of lifestyle: 1900–1980s

Geoffrey Rose's comments on the role of the population and the individual are taken from 'Strategy of Prevention: Lessons from Cardiovascular Disease', *British Medical Journal* 282 (1981): 1847–51. John Ryle's definition of social medicine is taken from J. A. Ryle, *Changing Disciplines* (London: Oxford University Press, 1948), pp. 11–12.

Chapter 6: Tropical and international public health

The comment about Africans is made in M. Vaughan, *Curing Their Ills: Colonial Power and African Illness* (Oxford: Polity Press, 1991), pp. 39–40.

The Ottawa Charter was published by the WHO in 1986.

The quote by John Manton is from 'Tropical Medicine' in V. Berridge, M. Gorsky, and A. Mold, eds, *Public Health in History* (Maidenhead: Open University Press, 2011), p. 83.

Chapter 7: Present and future in the light of history

The public health futures tale came from Martin O'Flaherty at the University of Liverpool and was published in the *Lancet* on 24 November 2014.

Peter Piot's comments were made during a Global Health Laboratory public meeting at the London School of Hygiene and Tropical Medicine in 2015.

The comment about confusion during the 2009 swine flu epidemic in England and fears of loss of independence is taken from my unpublished research on the epidemic carried out in 2010–11.

The reference to drug users' brains came from C. O'Brien, 'What Is Addiction and What Do Addictions Have in Common', plenary address to the Douglas Southall Freeman conference, 'Addictions Old and New', University of Richmond, Virginia, 22 October 2015.

Further reading

General

V. Berridge, M. Gorsky, and A. Mold, eds, *Public Health in History* (Maidenhead: Open University Press, 2011).

A.-E. Birn, Y. Pillay, and T. H. Holtz, eds, *Textbook of International Health: Global Health in a Dynamic World* (New York: Oxford University Press, 2009).

W. Bynum, *The History of Medicine: A Very Short Introduction* (Oxford: Oxford University Press, 2008).

R. Detels, R. Beaglehole, M. A. Lansing, and M. Gulliford, eds, *The Oxford Textbook of Public Health* (Oxford: Oxford University Press, 2009). Earlier editions are useful guides to both current and past public health. This version has an excellent historical article by Christopher Hamlin.

D. Porter, *Health, Civilisation and the State: A History of Public Health from Ancient to Modern Times* (London: Routledge, 1999).

D. Porter, ed., *The History of Public Health and the Modern State* (Amsterdam: Rodopi, 1994).

G. Rosen, *A History of Public Health*, expanded edition with introduction by Elizabeth Fee (Baltimore, MD: Johns Hopkins University Press, 1993), first published 1958.

C. Webster, ed., *Caring for Health: History and Diversity* (Buckingham: Open University Press, 2001).

books listed in the general section are useful, and also:

Baggott, *Public Health Policy and Politics*, 2nd ed. (Basingstoke: Palgrave Macmillan, 2011).

D. J. Hunter, *Public Health Policy* (Cambridge: Polity Press, 2003).

J. Lewis, *What Price Community Medicine? The Philosophy, Practice and Politics of Public Health Since 1919* (Brighton: Wheatsheaf, 1986).

T. McKeown, *The Role of Medicine: Dream, Mirage or Nemesis?* (Oxford: Blackwell, 1979).

Chapter 2: Current challenges

R. Beaglehole and R. Bonita, eds, *Global Public Health: A New Era*, 2nd ed. (Oxford: Oxford University Press, 2009). This contains many useful chapters, including those by A. McMichael and R. Beaglehole surveying the global context for public health, and by K. Lock and F. Sim on public health in the United Kingdom.

Commission on the Social Determinants of Health, *Closing the Gap in a Generation: Health Equity Through Action on the Social Determinants of Health. Final Report of the Commission on Social Determinants of Health* (Geneva: WHO, 2008).

D. Dorling, R. Mitchell, M. Shaw, S. Orford, and G. Davey Smith, 'The Ghost of Christmas Past: Health Effects of Poverty in London in 1896 and 1991', *British Medical Journal*, 321 (2000): 1547–51.

J. Hanefeld, ed., *Globalisation and Health* (Maidenhead: Open University Press, 2015).

S. Harman, *Global Health Governance* (London: Routledge, 2012).

R. Wilkinson and K. Pickett, *The Spirit Level: Why Equality Is Better for Everyone* (Harmondsworth: Penguin, 2010).

Chapter 3: The origins of public health into the 1700s

S. K. Cohn, *The Black Death Transformed: Disease and Culture in Early Modern Europe* (London: Arnold, 2001).

A. W. Crosby, *The Columbian Exchange: Biological and Cultural Consequences of 1492* (Westport, CT: Greenwood Publishing Company, 1972).

M. Harrison, *Contagion: How Commerce Has Spread Disease* (New Haven, CT, and London: Yale University Press, 2012).

V. Nutton, *Ancient Medicine* (London: Routledge, 2004).

C. Rawcliffe, *Urban Bodies: Communal Health in Late Medieval English Towns and Cities* (Woodbridge: The Boydell Press, 20...).

P. Slack, *Plague: A Very Short Introduction* (Oxford: Oxford Univer. Press, 2012).

Chapter 4: Sanitation to education: 1800–1900s

P. Baldwin, *Contagion and the State in Europe, 1830–1930* (Cambridge: Cambridge University Press, 1999).

J. Duffy, *The Sanitarians: A History of American Public Health* (Urbana: University of Illinois Press, 1990).

R. Evans, *Death in Hamburg: Society and Politics in the Cholera Years* (London: Penguin, 1987).

C. Hamlin, *Public Health and Social Justice in the Age of Chadwick: Britain, 1800–1854* (Cambridge: Cambridge University Press, 1998).

D. Kevles, *In the Name of Eugenics: Genetics and the Uses of Human Heredity* (Harmondsworth: Penguin, 1986).

A. La Berge, *Mission and Method: The Early Nineteenth-Century French Public Health Movement* (Cambridge: Cambridge University Press, 1992).

M. Worboys, *Spreading Germs: Disease Theories and Medical Practice in Britain, 1865–1900* (Cambridge: Cambridge University Press, 2000).

Chapter 5: The rise of lifestyle: 1900–1980s

V. Berridge, *AIDS in the UK: The Making of Policy, 1981–1994* (Oxford: Oxford University Press, 1996).

V. Berridge, *Marketing Health: Smoking and the Discourse of Public Health in Britain, 1945–2000* (Oxford: Oxford University Press, 2007).

V. Berridge and S. Blume, *Poor Health: Social Inequality Before and After the Black Report* (London: Frank Cass, 2003).

M. Honigsbaum, *Living With Enza: The Forgotten Story of Britain and the Great Flu Pandemic of 1918* (London and New York: Macmillan, 2009).

, M. Powell, J. Stewart, and B. Taylor, *Cradle to Grave: icipal Medicine in Interwar England and Wales* (Bern: Peter ig, 2011).

vis, *The Politics of Motherhood: Child and Maternal Welfare in ngland, 1900–1939* (London: Croom Helm, 1980).

Oppenheimer, 'Profiling Risk: The Emergence of Coronary Heart Disease Epidemiology in the United States, 1947–70', *International Journal of Epidemiology*, 35 (2006): 720–30.

W. G. Rothstein, *Public Health and the Risk Factor: A History of an Uneven Medical Revolution* (Rochester, NY: University of Rochester Press, 2003).

S. Szreter, 'The Importance of Social Intervention in Britain's Mortality Decline, c.1850–1914: A Re-interpretation of the Role of Public Health', *Social History of Medicine*, 1(1) (1988): 1–37.

J. Welshman, *Municipal Medicine: Public Health in Twentieth-Century Britain* (Oxford: Peter Lang, 2000).

Chapter 6: Tropical and international public health

S. Amrith, *Decolonising International Health: India and Southeast Asia, 1930–65* (Basingstoke: Palgrave, 2006).

W. Anderson, *Colonial Pathologies: American Tropical Medicine, Race and Hygiene in the Philippines* (Durham, NC: Duke University Press, 2006).

T. M. Brown, M. Cueto, and E. Fee, 'The World Health Organisation and the Transition from "International" to "Global" Public Health', *American Journal of Public Health*, 96(1) (2006): 62–72.

M. Cueto, 'The Origins of Primary Health Care and Selective Primary Health Care', *American Journal of Public Health*, 94(11) (2004): 1864–74.

P. Curtin, *Death by Migration: Europe's Encounter with the Tropical World in the Nineteenth Century* (Cambridge: Cambridge University Press, 1989).

M. Harrison, *Public Health in British India: Anglo-Indian Preventive Medicine, 1859–1914* (Cambridge: Cambridge University Press, 1994).

R. Iliffe, *The African AIDS Epidemic: A History* (Oxford: James Currey, 2006).

M. Lyons, *The Colonial Disease: A Social History of Sleeping Sickness in Northern Zaire, 1900–1940* (Cambridge: Cambridge University Press, 1992).

J. Manton, 'Tropical Medicine' and 'Global Health' in V. Berridge,
   M. Gorsky, and A. Mold, eds, *Public Health in History* pp. 74–89
   and 179–94 (Maidenhead: Open University Press, 2011).
R. Packard, *The Making of a Tropical Disease: A Short History of
   Malaria* (Baltimore, MD: Johns Hopkins University Press, 2007).
M. Vaughan, 'Syphilis in Colonial East and Central Africa: The Social
   Construction of an Epidemic' in T. Ranger and P. Slack, eds,
   *Epidemics and Ideas: Essays on the Historical Perception of
   Pestilence*, pp. 269–302 (Cambridge: Cambridge University Press,
   1992).
P. Weindling, *International Health Organisations and Movements,
   1918–1939* (Cambridge: Cambridge University Press, 1995).

Chapter 7: Present and future in the light of history

The influences on this chapter are too many to list in a bibliography,
   but some of the recent texts listed in the general section and for
   Chapter 2 will be useful.
The magazine published by the UK Faculty of Public Health, *Public
   Health Today*, covers national and some European and international
   issues in a readable way. The e-mail alerts of the American Public
   Health Association (APHA) throw light on public health issues
   from the US perspective.

Publisher's acknowledgements

We are grateful for permission to include the following copyright material in this book.

Extract on pp. 103–4 reprinted from *The Lancet*, 386, Naomi Lee, Pieter van de Graaf, Emma Hopkins, Martin O'Flaherty, 'Health of the UK population in 2040', pp. 643–4, Copyright 2015, with permission from Elsevier. http://www.sciencedirect.com/science/journal/01406736

The publisher and author have made every effort to trace and contact all copyright holders before publication. If notified, the publisher will be pleased to rectify any errors or omissions at the earliest opportunity.

Index

INFECTIOUS DISEASES

A Very Short Introduction

Marta L. Wayne and Benjamin Bolker

As doctors and biologists have learned, to their dismay, infectious disease is a moving target: new diseases emerge every year, old diseases evolve into new forms, and ecological and socioeconomic upheavals change the transmission pathways by which disease spread. By taking an approach focused on the general evolutionary and ecological dynamics of disease, this *Very Short Introduction* provides a general conceptual framework for thinking about disease. Through a series of case studies, Benjamin Bolker and Marta L. Wayne introduce the major ideas of infectious disease in a clear and thoughtful way, emphasising the general principles of infection, the management of outbreaks, and the evolutionary and ecological approaches that are now central to much research about infectious disease.

www.oup.com/vsi

...UGS

...y Short Introduction

...es Iversen

...twentieth century saw a remarkable upsurge of research
...drugs, with major advances in the treatment of bacterial and
...iral infections, heart disease, stomach ulcers, cancer, and
mental illnesses. These, along with the introduction of the oral
contraceptive, have altered all of our lives. There has also been an
increase in the recreational use and abuse of drugs in the Western
world. This *Very Short Introduction*, in its second edition, gives a
non-technical account of how drugs work in the body. Reviewing
both legal (alcohol, nicotine, and caffeine) and illegal drugs, Les
Iversen discusses why some are addictive, and whether drug
laws need reform.

EPIDEMIOLOGY
A Very Short Introduction
Rodolfo Saracci

Epidemiology has had an impact on many areas of medicine;
and lung cancer, to the origin and spread of new epidemics.
and lung cancer, to the origin and spread of new epidemics.
However, it is often poorly understood, largely due to
misrepresentations in the media. In this *Very Short Introduction*
Rodolfo Saracci dispels some of the myths surrounding the
study of epidemiology. He provides a general explanation of
the principles behind clinical trials, and explains the nature of
basic statistics concerning disease. He also looks at the ethical
and political issues related to obtaining and using information
concerning patients, and trials involving placebos.

MEDICAL LAW
A Very Short Introduction
Charles Foster

Medical law is concerned with our bodies, and what happens to them during and after our lives. When things go wrong with our bodies, we want to know what our rights are, and what governs the conduct of the clinicians into whose hands we put our lives and limbs. Dealing with matters of life and death, it can therefore have a fundamental impact on medical practice. Headlines in the media often involve the core issues of medical law - organ transplantation, abortion, withdrawal of treatment, euthanasia, confidentiality, research on humans - these are topics that affect us all. Headlines can misrepresent, however. In order to fully understand the issues and their relevance, we have to delve into the cases and into the principles behind them.

"colourful and engaging" - **Medical Law Review**